Might
Bite

Might Bite

The secret life of a gambling addict

Patrick Foster
with **Will Macpherson**

BLOOMSBURY SPORT
LONDON · OXFORD · NEW YORK · NEW DELHI · SYDNEY

BLOOMSBURY SPORT
Bloomsbury Publishing Plc
50 Bedford Square, London, WC1B 3DP, UK
29 Earlsfort Terrace, Dublin 2, Ireland

BLOOMSBURY, BLOOMSBURY SPORT and the Diana logo are trademarks of
Bloomsbury Publishing Plc

First published in Great Britain 2022

A catalogue record for this book is available from the British Library

ISBN: HB: 978-1-4729-9213-0; eBook: 978-1-4729-9214-7;
ePdf: 978-1-4729-9215-4

2 4 6 8 10 9 7 5 3 1

Typeset in Minion Pro by Deanta Global Publishing Services, Chennai, India
Printed and bound in Great Britain by CPI Group (UK) Ltd, Croydon CR0 4YY

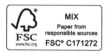

To find out more about our authors and books visit www.bloomsbury.com
and sign up for our newsletters

CONTENTS

FOREWORD BY MARCUS TRESCOTHICK

I first met Patrick Foster in October 2018 at the Oval Cricket Ground in south London. We were sat in the grand old Committee Room inside the historic Pavilion, launching the Professional Cricketers' Trust, a charity that supports players of our great game, past and present.

The two of us had been invited to tell our stories to print and broadcast media, thus raising awareness of the Trust's amazing work. Patrick and I had been asked to speak together because we had very different experiences in cricket and in life.

At the Oval 12 years earlier, I had played the last of my 76 Test matches for England. A dozen years on, I had just completed the 26th of my 27 years as a professional with Somerset. Cricket had given me a great life and livelihood.

In his teens and early twenties, Patrick had also been a professional cricketer with Northamptonshire, playing nine first-class matches for Durham University. It had been his dream to make a career from the game, as I did.

But things had not gone quite to plan, and he had spent the decade before we met getting a degree, working in insurance and teaching while being an outstanding club cricketer. Cricket was a big part of his life, but he had done much else besides.

So as professional cricketers we had a lot of differences, but we were also sat talking to each other and telling our stories because as people, we had much in common. We had both had battles with mental health. My issue had been depression, triggered particularly by travelling away from home while under the intense spotlight of being an international cricketer. Patrick's was a pathological addiction to gambling that caused many other problems. We were both cricketers who had had major struggles off the field.

Just a few months before we met, Patrick had been totally gripped by his addiction, which drove him right to the brink. But in that room he told his incredible story with clarity and calm. It was raw and tough to hear, but it was compulsive listening. I had said my bit, a tale which many in the room knew well, then everyone was gripped by Patrick's story, even though most there did not know too much about him. Speaking about such matters so soon after they had happened takes a bit of courage. I was sat there thinking that this was someone who had been pushed to some extraordinary lengths and been to some dark places, beyond his control. Given what we had in common, it really hit home.

We were both there, too, because we were so grateful for the support we had received from the Professional Cricketers' Association, the parent body of the PCT. In 2006 I had come home from a tour of India having suffered a breakdown, and the help – through counselling – I received was instant and impressive. Just having someone I could sit down and open up to, who made me feel I was not alone was so powerful. The PCA had helped Patrick in his recovery, and we both felt so lucky to have them.

Now, Patrick works with them. Back in 2018, he was learning how to tell his story, and taking the first steps in a new life. The words he was saying were raw, and incredible to hear. These days, the narrative is polished and professional, but no less affecting. It makes for harrowing listening, that I found I could really relate to. It does not make for easy listening, but it is also amazing to see him stood there before you – or, in the pandemic, at the other end of a screen! – in recovery.

He speaks to students at schools and universities around the country, and to every professional cricketer (man and woman) in the country through the PCA, as well as plenty of other people across the sporting sphere.

He is sharing such an important message. Since he opened up about his struggles, another professional cricketer, Hampshire's Chris Wood, has come forward and told his own story, and now they work together, which is very good to see. There are more young people in cricket who need help with gambling, and these two are doing a great job helping them. Patrick is a trailblazer because every person who talks about their experiences makes it easier for the next.

One of the things about problem gambling that has struck me since hearing Patrick's story and learning that Chris – who I played against a lot – had a problem, is how little education there has been around it. I certainly wasn't warned of gambling's dangers growing up and I probably made it halfway through my career as a cricketer before it was ever raised as a 'problem', whereas we were in no doubt that drink or drugs could cause trouble. Over the years I have seen plenty of players gamble in many different ways, and they need to know that it can spiral out of control, as it did for Patrick.

As a society, it feels we are only just getting to grips with gambling addiction. It is not as normalised as other mental health struggles. Now this taboo is being smashed, we can move on to the next.

But I do believe we are fostering an easier environment for people to open up, whatever their issues. I look at some of the young cricketers I work with, like Dom Bess, a former teammate of mine at Somerset is in his early twenties. He has already learnt to speak articulately about his battles with his mental health, and that will help others. People across sport and society are just so much more ready to express their feelings, to ask for help.

I wrote extensively about my depression in 2008 in my book *Coming Back To Me*. It was a cathartic process, but also hard because I was still an active cricketer and learning how to deal with my mental health.

I am very proud to have played a part in opening up the conversation, and – hopefully – allowing more people to get help. I have said before that I wrote that book thinking that if I helped one person feel better in the battle I had been fighting, I would be happy. It would all be worth it. Fortunately, many people have said over the years that it helped them. And, honestly, I am as proud of my role in that conversation as I am of any cricketing achievement – a cap, a hundred, a series win. I'm extremely proud to see other cricketers – like Jonathan Trott, Steve Harmison, Mike Yardy and Sarah Taylor – opening up about their mental health. Cricketers and sportspeople are more vulnerable than they might first appear.

My time as a cricketer was great, I loved it and feel so lucky. But like all things, it came to an end. For me this was in 2019, when I began another chapter on the other side of the boundary as a coach, first with Somerset and now with England.

But education on all matters mental health keeps going. It is a lifelong project. I still get a buzz talking about it, helping people, making the sort of appearance at which I met Patrick. I find this work endures far more than runs or wickets. I am proud that Patrick is on the same path. His work will help many.

1

March 2018

Having driven around aimlessly for three hours, I left my car at Slough station and didn't bother to pay for parking. Instead, having earlier smashed a porcelain piggybank I shared with my girlfriend and taken what I thought was my final £18.10, I bought a ticket to London, and walked onto the platform. The departures board told me that in six minutes a train would be hurtling through without stopping. I was set on throwing myself in front of it.

Standing on the end of the platform, I was certain that, despite only having turned 31 three days earlier, I'd reached the end of the road. I was ready to end my total mess of a life. I'd experienced suicidal thoughts for some time, and this was my second attempt to take my life in the course of 12 extraordinary days that had pushed me to the point of no return.

Although things had come to a head in 12 days, in reality they had been building up over the previous 12 years. In that time I'd developed a secret gambling addiction that had caused me trouble and pain in ways I could never have imagined. It had crippled me emotionally and financially, and it had led to me lying so much and so often that I became a master of disguise, living a double life.

To others, I was Patrick (or 'Patch'), the life and soul of the party. I was a hard-working professional. I was a former professional cricketer who remained fanatical about playing and watching sport. I was from a happy, supportive family. I was a strong partner to a brilliant girlfriend. I was generally a well-rounded young man with plenty going for me and even more to look forward to. Certainly not perfect, but who is?

In reality, I was angry, saddled with debt and carrying a dirty secret that not even those closest to me knew. I'd become a fine liar and actor, able to put on a brave face, even when things were going very, very wrong.

People knew I liked a punt. Some knew it had got me into the occasional scrape. But gambling had become the defining aspect of my personality – and no one else knew that. I gambled at every opportunity. And because I gambled, I lied, sometimes about unthinkable topics, and I stole. I stole from those close to me, and from those I barely knew. I stole money intended for charity.

I always drank, but at times, because I gambled, I descended into alcoholism and dabbled with drugs. Because I gambled, I suffered from anxiety, depression and stress so severe it gave me a stomach ulcer.

Often, as soon as the door shut and I was alone, I would simply break down in tears. I was so, so tired of lying, yet I barely slept through the night for seven years; I would be awake indulging my addiction, or dealing with its devastating consequences. The first and last things I thought of on each long day weren't my loved ones, but gambling.

I couldn't stop gambling. Across these 12-and-a-half years, I placed just shy of £2m in online bets, and probably the same again in betting shops and casinos.

In March 2018 I had 19 different accounts with online bookmakers. At my peak, in 2017, I'd had 76 accounts in 65 different names. I was a VIP member of seven different online operators; in most cases, I had to be spending a minimum of £30,000 per year to qualify.

I'd received close to £110,000 in free bets. That year, 2017, I placed 27,988 bets with a single bookmaker. That's close to 77 bets every day – and that's just with one bookie.

There was nothing I wouldn't bet on. I'd always been passionate about cricket, football, golf and rugby union – particularly when they involved British players and teams. From the word go I loved the thrill of watching a roulette wheel spin.

But I became less and less fussy. I gambled on Hungarian handball, considered myself an expert on American horse racing from Santa Anita, California, and even found myself gripped by Ecuadorian U23 football in the early hours of the morning. I once won close to £20,000 on a basketball accumulator based on the number of points scored in each game, despite not having heard of any of the teams, let alone players, involved. In the course of that very night I lost every penny of the win, predicting which team was going to score the next try and whether the conversion would be missed in an Australian rugby league game between Cronulla Sharks and South Sydney Rabbitohs. Knowledge or informed judgements ceased to matter – I just needed to bet.

That need, though, overwhelmed me and, because I couldn't speak about it, made me feel like I was being eaten from the inside out. I'd locked my issues away, but the walls were closing in every single day until finally there was no way out.

I was always convinced that I could bet my way out of trouble and move on with my life. The belief that gambling would be my escape from gambling was naturally one of the many reasons I did so much of it.

Yet there were occasions when I won big enough amounts to erase my debts and walk away. At one stage in 2016 I had more than £96,000 across my many online gambling accounts – enough to get me out of trouble, but not enough to satisfy my addiction: I always wanted more. If I had £96,000, why not tick it into six figures? But that wouldn't have been enough either. I was greedy and had lost all sense of money's value. A few days later I lost it all and was back to square one, scratching around until my next payday.

Owning up to ease the pain? That never felt like much of an option. I responded to every moment of adversity in my adult life, not by talking to others and working through my problems, but by bottling bad feelings away and falling back on the thing that comforted me – gambling.

I was too proud and too fearful of the consequences to reveal my quandary, and continued to be suffocated by its weight and ever-deepening nature. I needed help but I felt that telling anyone – my lovely girlfriend, my adoring family or supportive mates – would come at too much of a cost. I would lose everything, and I couldn't bear that.

By now, I'd lost almost everything anyway. That day, I was due to learn that a career I loved was over. At 31, I was becoming a former teacher, and in a shameful fashion. At 24, I'd become a former insurance broker. And at 20, I'd become a former professional cricketer. The loss of all three careers, each more than the last, was due to my gambling.

I'd no money left. In fact – I'd much less than that. My gambling led to me living way beyond my means, and I'd supplemented my teacher's salary – which had averaged about £32,000 per year in my time in the job – in increasingly desperate ways. I'd taken out 23 bank, payday or unsecured loans. I'd borrowed money from loan sharks and drug dealers. I'd borrowed money from the parents of children I'd taught, and from colleagues. I'd borrowed money from friends and family. In total, since my gambling began, I'd borrowed money from 113 different people, adding up to £497,000. The necessity to repay some of these loans and the odd hefty win meant not all of this was debt. That said, I still had £238,000 outstanding, that was effectively due to be repaid immediately.

In the week since my last suicide attempt, my situation had worsened, my despair had deepened and my conviction had grown much stronger: I saw no other way out.

*　　*　　*

The final descent began when, 12 days earlier, I received an email that made me lie awake all that night, racked with anxiety. It was from a parent of a kid I taught whom I'd previously borrowed a significant amount of money from. He was asking why the repayments had dried up and, frankly, what on earth was going on? This inquiry had been triggered by a conversation with another parent, from whom I'd also borrowed money. The two of them had realised they were not alone. The email very pointedly questioned whether my issue was, in fact, gambling. If it was, he said, that made the whole thing worse, and he'd have no choice but to inform the school.

I was terrified. I'd never been questioned like this before. I knew that if he did tell the school, then my fabricated life would unravel. I tried to quell his obvious anger by assuring him that I would sort out his repayments as soon as possible.

To make things worse, late the previous week I'd also made other desperate requests for financial help to people I should have known not to contact. In general, their response was to reply with concern, not only about the content of my messages but the tone. A number of them said they couldn't keep it to themselves. I felt like my house of cards was about to fall.

I'd been in trouble at school before, notably over an incident involving damage to a school minibus that I'd worsened by lying about – brazenly and at length, meaning the whole thing rumbled on and became far uglier than it could have been. I'd denied any wrongdoing when I was clearly the only person who could have been the culprit. Lying and running away from problems were second nature to me.

And that was before we even came to the lying, borrowing and misbehaviour that was directly linked to my life as a secret gambling addict, all of which was yet to come to light. For some time, my desperation to gamble had seen me abuse my authority as a teacher; in the case of some of the most significant loans I'd taken from people, a little had been paid back. But now I had defaulted on almost all the repayments.

So I woke up on Monday morning very nervous. The more I thought about the email, the more fearful I became that the parent was going to tell the school. I couldn't think about anything else. I'd become extremely paranoid that the hundreds of skeletons in my closet would be exposed, and I went into panic mode. I knew I was skating on thin ice, and had so much to lose. The job, obviously. But also, the house I lived in with my girlfriend, which was paid for by the school. The scale of my offences meant that surely I would be stripped of my right to teach, taken to court for fraud and possibly even sent to prison. I needed to find a way to get this man – and the many others – his money back. If he did expose me, it would be the beginning of the end.

More than any formal punishment, the consequence that filled me with the most dread was my actions becoming public, and having to explain myself to my friends and family. Rather than act rationally by seeking advice (I now realise, looking back, that any advice, legal or personal, would have done), I chose to gamble. It was my safety net and the only coping mechanism I felt I had left. And I believed there was still one last route out of this extraordinary mess – the Cheltenham Festival, which was due to start the following day. Cheltenham is a four-day horse racing meet in Gloucestershire with the best jump horses, the biggest prize money, and the eyes of the racing world on it. All the opportunity it promised made it heaven for me. It was my favourite time of the year and it had been on my mind for weeks. It was my final shot at salvation.

The trouble was, I'd gambled all my money away, and so needed to find some more, by whatever means I could. My account was empty, and payday was still more than a fortnight away. And anyway, when that payday arrived, it would go on the tens of thousands of pounds I owed in loan repayments. But by now, this sort of quandary wasn't something that fazed me.

I persuaded one of my many VIP managers at an online bookmaker to give me £100 in free bets, and I sold a couple of tickets I had for the Thursday of the Festival to a friend of a friend for a good whack – £300. The tickets had been a freebie from another gambling company. They lavish their biggest losers – those who gamble the most – with compensatory gifts. Profiting from something I had been given for free didn't bother me in the slightest.

And then came a phone call. As someone with two lives, I hated phone calls, preferring to communicate via WhatsApp or email because it was less personal and easier to run away from or block out. But this was urgent, and I was really desperate.

I'd exhausted all avenues for ready cash at my current school, so went back to a figure I respected greatly and had borrowed from before. This person was extremely wealthy, extremely generous, and was someone with whom I'd developed a great relationship over time. They had said that, were I ever in trouble, I should get in touch again. As a bonus, there was next to no possibility of a chance encounter in the coming days.

Feeling this wasn't an opportunity I could pass up, I went for broke – in excruciating fashion. I explained in some detail how a close family member had received some devastating news about their health. Their chances of survival were slim and relied on urgent treatment that would come at significant cost when done privately. The cost, I said, was £10,000 but that I would be able to pay the loan back in a week, when the surgery was done and my family member was able to access their funds.

Not a word of this was true and my real belief, of course, was that I would be able to pay this person – and countless others, including the man badgering me – back when Cheltenham was over and I'd completed the simple task of turning 10 grand into 150 grand, which was the figure I thought would get me out of trouble at school and therefore spare me jail. I'd won big before. Easy.

They asked to consider for a few hours, which I spent in a state of overwhelming anxiety, keeping a low profile at school, constantly refreshing my emails, and gambling away that free bet I'd been given. Just before 5 p.m., this person came through, sending the money on the terms agreed on the phone. Flooded with relief, I could scarcely believe it.

Then came a period of intense study: working out how I would use my pot. I opted to be consistent in who I backed, choosing the Gigginstown House Stud, the trainer Gordon Elliott and the jockey Davy Russell. I wouldn't back them exclusively, but they would be the focus of my more elaborate bets.

Tuesday and Wednesday? A blur. I tried to balance teaching, gambling, and watching what I was gambling on – which, by the way, wasn't just Cheltenham, but racing at Fontwell Park, cricket in the Pakistan Super League and, in the evening, any football that was on. I finished each day off with a trip to the virtual casino.

There were some early wins, but they tailed off. I was increasingly despondent, feeling physically sick and, by Thursday morning, ready to give up. I had only about £2,000 of the loan left, but it felt like a full-time job keeping tabs on how much I'd lost across all 19 accounts, and what I'd actually bet on.

Each morning at work, waiting for the racing to begin, was a greater test of resolve than the last – especially because I felt like a marked man by senior staff and feared every parent. It felt like everyone was looking at me, and I kept a very low profile, hiding myself away and avoiding communal areas. Thursday was my half-day, so I headed to the pub to watch the racing and drown my sorrows in the company of the landlord, who also liked a flutter.

Earlier that day, during a free period, I'd placed a series of bets based on a hunch that this would be a good day for the Irish and for Gordon Elliott. Among them was a 'Lucky 15', which is among the most complicated bets available, but is familiar to the seasoned gambler. It includes four single bets, six doubles (in a double, you bet on two outcomes and need both to be successful), four trebles (in a treble, you bet on three outcomes and need all of them to be successful) and a four-fold (in a four-fold, also known as a quadruple, you bet on four outcomes and need all of them to be successful) across four different events. Each of the above bets stand in isolation, however with every win, the odds for the next bet increase, and the final selection is worth double odds from the outset. My stake was £2 (so a total of £30 across the 15 bets), and I backed a few of my selections in extra standalone bets too, just in case. I thought nothing more of it as over the years I'd made hundreds of bets with such seemingly insignificant stakes that were all very unlikely to come good.

But slowly, they started coming in... Shattered Love, ridden by Will Kennedy and trained by Gordon Elliott, roared home and the landlord – who had copied that bet – appeared with his arms aloft. Then Delta Work, a French horse ridden by Davy Russell and trained by Gordon Elliott, did the same. So too Balko Des Flos, defeating a massive favourite (I'd also backed the favourite as a contingency). I was in complete shock.

Having calmed myself down using the tried and tested combination of Stella Artois and Marlboro Lights, my fourth horse, Storyteller, won the 4.10. My £30 stake had returned £28,672.60. Not only that, but I'd backed all four separately. When I staggered home an hour later, I had won about £58,000 across my 19 different online accounts. That was getting on for double my annual salary.

I spent the evening with my girlfriend Charlotte, who had been hard at work during the day. I pretended nothing had happened – and as far as she was concerned, nothing had. I wasn't celebrating wildly, as so many would be. Any right-minded person would have been delighted to win £58,000, which was more than enough to get myself out of a lot of trouble and clear plenty of debts – especially the very urgent ones.

Instead, my thinking was that I was still in deep trouble, and this big win only partially alleviated that. Time was running out, in every sense. The Festival had just one day left and I was still a long way from where I wanted to be. I needed to clear all my debts, not just the most pressing ones.

I was also convinced that every second that passed brought me closer to oblivion at school. I'd convinced myself that I was the last to know that I was being investigated, or fired. I had to keep going. The stress was wearing me down – and it had taken its toll on my physical appearance, too. I was massively overweight and I was so tired that only caffeine tablets washed down with coffee kept me on my feet.

I woke up on Friday morning hungover, and the stomach ulcer – for which I was taking daily medication – was searingly painful. My paranoia and anxiety surged once more. The morning was a mighty struggle.

Friday at Cheltenham is Gold Cup Day, the biggest event of the Festival. Historically, I'd put more money on this race than any other in the calendar. I'd enjoyed great success at times but also some crushing losses. It also represented a kind of anniversary, harking back to some brilliant days out, getting smashed with mates.

I'd known for some time who I was backing in the biggest race: Might Bite. A year earlier, I saw this horse win after I'd backed it heavily in a two-part bet that saw the first horse lose.

I felt this was a moment for redemption. It was meant to be. I was so certain that I'd already placed some early bets when the £10,000 loan had come in at the start of the week.

The early part of the day went awfully, and I was down about £18,000 by the time I glumly entered the classroom for a lesson at 3 p.m. – the graveyard shift. In the moments before the kids came into the room, I bet everything I had in my 19 accounts on Might Bite. I'd also popped into two local bookies that afternoon in a free period. In total, I'd put almost £50,000 on this horse to win at odds of 7/2 and 10/3.

Having felt sick for days, everything suddenly seemed quite simple. If Might Bite and jockey Nico de Boinville won, I would win just over £200,000, meaning I could pay off the £152,000 that I owed to those connected to the school, which would at least stop me going to jail. The rest? I could give that to my parents as an apology for letting them down so badly.

If it lost, I would have nothing, and very little option but to kill myself.

The boys filed into the classroom and I set them a Common Entrance mock examination. Instructions were on the board and the kids, aged 12 and 13, were immaculately behaved. They sat in silence, I sat at my desk and, on the computer in front of me, watched the most important three miles and two-and-a-half furlongs of my life.

In this silent room, they were off. Other horses fell, and this quickly became a two-horse race, a battle between my horse, Might Bite, and Native River. I just watched, without commentary, as the boys scribbled their answers, barely making a peep. I was just about sentient enough to appreciate that this was a classic battle between two great horses, lengths in front of the rest. Native River led for much of the race, but as they crossed the final fences, Might Bite stayed as close as can be. It was brilliant sport.

As Native River pulled away in the final stages to win by four-and-a-half lengths, and the jockey Richard Johnson raised his whip in celebration, I calmly clicked the little red cross in the corner of my screen to exit the browser. This was one of the greatest races in recent memory. Jumping the last fence, it had looked for all the world like Might Bite would outlast his rival. It wasn't to be. The silence in the classroom was eerie.

My reaction was one of acceptance and realisation rather than devastation or despondency. I felt numb. The game was up. I walked to the back of the classroom and stared out of the window for the final 20 minutes of the lesson, contemplating what came next. Time stood still.

That was that, then. The boys left the classroom and I slowly packed my things away, considering the simplest way to do a very difficult thing: kill myself. I'd considered driving my car off the road, or taking every pill I could get my hands on.

Instead, I left school and, rather than head home, set off towards Slough. I'd identified a position between Slough and Windsor where a bridge lay above the main line to London. I pulled up the car, and dangled my legs over the edge of the bridge. I sat there for about 90 minutes, crying and contemplating how I had reached this point.

Could I throw myself over the edge? I'd said goodbye to nobody, I'd not written a note. Yet I still had things I needed to say. I would find out any day now whether I was actually in trouble or not; perhaps that would help me find a way out. Maybe the problems would even just drift away. On Tuesday, it was my birthday, and Charlotte had gone to all sorts of trouble and expense arranging plans with my family over the weekend. And it was term time, and something like this would send shockwaves through a small community that meant a lot to me, even if I had not been treating it that way.

I desperately wanted to jump but I wasn't ready, and the timing just wasn't right. I slowly returned home, got in the bath, and cried some more, waiting for Charlotte to return from work. By the time she did, I'd put on the brave face that I'd used so often.

I didn't slip out of that mode for a few days. I spent the weekend with my family and friends, enjoying their company and being wined and dined. I had a lovely time, and no one thought anything was wrong. Occasionally I sloped off for a moment alone and the emotion poured out. But I resolved not to do anything, or tell anyone anything, just yet.

I would have found myself in an awkward predicament had I needed to pay for anything, but I didn't. As so often, I'd persuaded a mate of mine to lend me a few quid to tide me over, but I didn't want to spend it. I was, though, able to place a few bets because the bookies had made such a killing out of me on Friday that they dished out a few more free bets. They came to nothing. The bets I placed were completely far-fetched and hopeless. They were accumulators (one bet made up of multiple selections combined, and all the selections must win). These particular accumulators had very low stakes and very long odds. If they came through, they might get me out of trouble. But I didn't think for a second they would. Winning felt impossible now.

I hadn't felt like celebrating my birthday at all, but went through the motions. Charlotte was incredible again, buying me flights to Amsterdam, where I'd never been before, in May, and showering me with gifts. When I opened her card, my guard dropped. While she was touched that I showed so much emotion on learning of the surprise, I was inconsolable, riddled with guilt and shame.

At school, I was extremely paranoid – colleagues seemed to be talking about me. This was especially true on Wednesday evening, the night before term ended, when staff hosted a quiz for the boarders with all sorts of fun rounds to keep them entertained. I'd been actively avoiding my colleagues but now needed to show my face because I really had no choice. What I witnessed unsettled me deeply. Various senior members of staff were marching around having very serious-looking conversations with other, more junior members of staff. Those being quizzed were almost all good mates of mine or people whose money I'd 'borrowed'. I couldn't escape the feeling that I was the subject of their conversations. I asked mates but was told not to worry about it. Later on, everyone went to the pub and I was so paranoid that I started texting people, following up my earlier questions. Deep down, I knew I'd been found out.

I was absolutely dreading Thursday, the last day of term, for two reasons. One, because I was certain that the end of term would be a convenient time for the school to call me in for a meeting that would instigate the collapse of everything. But also because my attempts to avoid everyone would have to end. For weeks, lots of staff members had booked to go and play footgolf (a combination of football and golf where you kick a football into a big golf hole), which would also involve drinking punishments for poor performance. I'd helped make this into a bit of a tradition at this time of year – it was partly for my birthday, and partly because it was the end of term. I could hardly pull out.

After another night of no sleep, Thursday arrived. My predictions proved right. After breakfast, the boys were due to leave. A colleague found me, and told me that he'd just seen the Head and I was being summoned for a meeting. When they asked what it could be about, I laughed it off and acted surprised but I knew full well what was coming. As I'd suspected, my world was coming crashing down.

I was informed by the Acting Head and the Head of HR that the school had received complaints from the parent body regarding money – borrowing from parents of kids I taught, and failing to repay them.

The school said they had been conducting an official investigation into my behaviour and that I would be invited back for another meeting in due course, to which I would be able to bring a family member, a lawyer, a union representative or a colleague. I came from a family full of teachers and had plenty of mates in the industry, so I would have had a number of strong candidates, but I was beyond caring. I laughed the suggestion off.

At this stage, they didn't tell me what the outcome would be if they found me guilty – although I knew full well that what I'd done meant that it was just a matter of time before they did so. The investigation, I was told, would take some time, but the Easter holidays allowed them the opportunity to complete it.

It wasn't hard to know what the basic consequences would be, though. My job was surely gone and with it went my house. It seemed certain to me that there would be legal and perhaps criminal proceedings too, with the Teaching Regulation Authority certain to be involved. I again thought I would end up in prison.

I was left in no doubt about the gravity of the situation, and how thorough the investigation would be. It was the end of term, so I wasn't officially suspended from my job, but there was, to my mind, one good bit of news: I was no longer allowed to go on a school trip to Europe's battlefields that was leaving on Friday, the following day. I'd been dreading it, so this was music to my ears.

For the rest of the meeting, I was numb and barely able to focus on what was being said. There was no point paying attention when there seemed no use carrying on. My mind was made up. I hardly responded to what they said.

When I walked out, a car full of mates was waiting for me, beers in hand. I'd hoped to slink off home and gather my thoughts. But why not join them? It was certainly easier. My problems could wait a few hours. And if I was going to kill myself, I might as well have some fun before I did so.

These mates were my colleagues, and word now really had got around about my meeting so I was getting questions from all angles. When we arrived, I explained that I'd fucked up, things would become clear in the coming days, but it had nothing to do with the kids. There seemed to be some respect from the group that I'd addressed it, and it wasn't mentioned again – to me, at least. By then, I'd desperately asked one of my closest colleagues to borrow £200 to get through the day, and he'd obliged.

I proceeded to get extremely drunk, putting away plenty of cans of Stella. I wasn't worried about returning to the flat, because Charlotte, still completely unaware of how her long-term partner's life had fallen apart, was staying with her mum, as she sometimes did, to shorten her commute, and because I was due to head off on the Europe trip the following day.

It was still only early afternoon, but I wasn't in a good way when we returned to the village after footgolf. I still had £100 and a few coins remaining in my wallet. I got some food with the coins, then went to Coral in anticipation of placing my last-ever bet. I stuck all £100 on a horse called King Crimson, ridden by one of my favourite jockeys, Adam Kirby, in the 2.10 at Wolverhampton. I watched it come fourth – having led most of the way – with the betting slip already crumpled in my hand. What now?

I went home and smashed the piggy bank that Charlotte, rather than me, had put change in for us to save. I furiously picked up the £18.10, disappointed there was so little there. In my rage, I marched to the pub, and informed the landlord that I'd lost my wallet – another lie. I asked for a tab and told him I would pay it off the following day. I sat there for hours, stepping out only for a cigarette. I continued to get absolutely smashed as if nothing was happening. Eventually, I headed home and passed out fully clothed on the kitchen floor, among the smashed porcelain of the piggy bank.

On Friday morning, I woke late, colossally hungover and completely dazed, to a concerned message from Charlotte (who thought I was on the school trip). I'd also received a voicemail and an email from my dad, asking me to call him urgently. This wasn't good news; my dad was an experienced and respected headmaster at another school and we inhabited a small world. Who had told him what I'd done?

No one, exactly. But several of my friends had contacted him expressing concern that I was asking for money. I gave Dad short shrift and told him I would discuss it the following week, when we were due to see one another again. I knew the game was up.

I walked into the bathroom and collected every single pill we had in the house. There was a mix of antidepressants, sleeping pills, and treatment for my stomach ulcer – 97 in total. I took a load, then manically googled what would happen if I took the lot. When I couldn't find a clear answer, I kicked over the table they sat on and stormed out of the house.

I just started driving around the local streets, looking for any opportunity to rid myself of the pain I was experiencing. I drove for a couple of hours, finally pulling up at Slough station and walking solemnly to the end of platform 5.

I just had six minutes to wait.

2

October 2006

Lying in the bed of my dingy room in student halls, it's safe to say the last thing I needed was to be disturbed. I was still wearing my socks from the night before, and my head was pounding after too many Vodka-Red Bulls. My memory, at best, was hazy – what had I done to embarrass myself this time?

I was awoken from my slumber by two ominous, familiar sounds: creaking floorboards and cackling blokes, recounting the previous night's events. The sound edged closer, until this group of alpha males – my new mates, all cut from the same cloth as me – barged into my mess of a room like a swarm of unwanted wasps. It felt inevitable that they would suggest a trip to the local Lloyds No. 1 Bar for a full English and hair of the dog that had become customary in such situations over the previous couple of weeks as we all settled into freshers' life.

The lads had other ideas, though. They were off to the bookies. Feeling like death warmed up, I was taken aback and pleasantly surprised that more alcohol wouldn't immediately be consumed, prising myself out of bed and throwing on some tracksuit bottoms and the nearest hoody. We made tracks, via Greggs, for breakfast, coffee and a large bottle of water, with all the chat about the day's football.

We arrived at our destination, a Coral bookies, and my mates barged through the door. I followed, excited. I was 19, and had never stepped foot in a bookmakers before. In fact, I'd only had the most limited dealings with gambling. Occasionally, when we returned to Kenya – where my dad used to work and I was born – he would pop into a casino after an evening out to back his favourite number 29 on the roulette table while enjoying a nightcap.

And annually, we would have a family flutter on the Grand National. Every year, in April, my family and sometimes friends would gather round the TV and watch 40 horses thrash around four miles, two-and-a-half furlongs and the small matter of 30 fences. Earlier in the day I would've cut the names and silks of the competing jockeys out of the newspaper, we would all make a selection, then Dad would make his way into the nearest village to place a £5 bet for each of us. These seemingly insignificant stakes would be placed on horses that we, like so many others across the country, had chosen simply on the basis of their colours and names.

So, after an exciting build-up, the race would follow roughly the same pattern. Mum would ask over and over which horse was hers, but end up taking home a few quid. My brother would be convinced his horse would win because it approached the first hurdle in the lead. My dad was barely able to watch because, after all, this was his money, which he'd ultimately wasted as the horse he'd backed to win came second. My sister would be left devastated by the trail of destruction, with horses falling left, right and centre. One of those falling horses would inevitably be mine, so all that excitement would turn to anti-climax. And that would be that for another 12 months.

So, stepping into Coral, I knew next to nothing about gambling. I was entering a world that was entirely unfamiliar. It was a hub of activity, an eclectic and extraordinary mix of young and old, rich and poor, all there for their own reasons on a freezing morning in October, in the heart of the beautiful cathedral city of Durham.

My mates knew rather better what they were doing, striding towards the shop's corner to collect a form for their 'accumulator' and a tiny blue plastic biro. As they nattered about home and away records in the Vauxhall Conference, I watched a middle-aged man constantly feeding £20 notes into a Fixed Odds Betting Terminal (FOBT) to play online roulette. After 10 minutes, he hit the machine like a heavyweight boxer in a fit of rage and, with a cigarette lit before he was out the door, stormed onto the street and towards the nearest ATM. I watched this debacle unfold with a chuckle and, as I took my place in his still-warm swivelling bucket chair, thought what an idiot he must be.

I was out of my depth, but this did feel different to my very limited previous experiences of gambling; this was my time and money. I wanted to find out what the fuss was about for myself, and there was only one thing I was ever going to do. I scrambled around in my pocket, locating the two £1 coins I'd been given as change in Greggs and put them into the machine.

On a roulette board, zero is green, the only number that is not red or black. It had been the last number to come up, the one that had forced my predecessor to march out of the shop. The odds of zero coming up twice in a row are 1,369/1, but so what? I was 19, privileged, somewhere on the hazy border between confident and arrogant, and very fortunate. So my £2 went on green zero and I whacked the big red start button like a US President declaring nuclear war. Twelve seconds later, a small silver ball-bearing nestled itself in the bed of green zero. These were 12 seconds that changed my life forever.

After some deliberation, I showed some (brief) wisdom, perhaps based on events I'd just seen in this shop, and collected my winnings. As I walked over to the plastic screens on the other side of the shop, I had a beaming smile on my face. I collected my £72 from Angie behind the perspex; little did I know that I would get to know this woman, and many like her, extremely well.

I wandered back to rejoin my mates, bragging that I'd just paid for last night's entertainment with the click of a button. Following their lead, I reinvested £2 of the £72 back into an 18-game football accumulator, from which I stood to win close to £300,000. All I needed was Sheffield Wednesday to win away at Leeds United, Crystal Palace to sneak a draw with West Bromwich Albion, and many other results to go my way. Like everyone else, I was adamant that this was going to happen.

We left the shop, with our hangovers easing and a spring in our step for the afternoon ahead. After a brief con-flab outside the shop, some went off to do battle on the college rugby fields, some to see their latest girlfriend, and others to further nurse their hangovers.

Not me, though. I watched the others walk off before executing a perfect 180 and headed straight back into the shop. After all, I had £70 that I'd done nothing to earn. Why not try turn it into £700?

As I re-entered just a few minutes after walking out, most of those inside had barely moved an inch. On the TV, Jeff Stelling was starting his weekly broadcast of *Soccer Saturday*. On screens around him were some One-Day International cricket matches in India, some South African horse racing at the Vaal and some virtual horse racing at Sprint Valley (virtual racing, it turns out, is computerised racing set up entirely to offer gamblers an opportunity to bet in the absence of actual racing; Sprint Valley is one of their made-up venues). All of it suddenly looked very appealing.

My intention was to pop in and check if Hibernian were leading in the early kick-off, as I needed them to win for my accumulator. The reality was that I got settled in what felt like splendid isolation. There were others in the shop, of course, but everyone was happily gambling away in their own little bubble.

As the greyhounds emerged from their traps, the horses gathered at the start and footballers made their way out through the tunnels I found myself leaving the bucket chair in front of the roulette machine and visiting Angie to make regular reinvestments. Some won, some lost, some fell and some simply romped home, but this fun new game felt like it was built for me.

Not only that, but I loved the venue too. I was obsessed with sport. I had been my whole adult life. By the age of 10, like many young kids, I was just a sponge for sports knowledge. I'd watch anything that happened to be on TV. I loved cricket and rugby, which I played so much of. I wasn't that into football because I didn't go to schools that played the game but had supported Liverpool vaguely since I first moved over from Kenya as a kid. My best mate supported Sheffield United and took me to watch them. I chose to support their opponents.

The amount of time I spent watching sport, or talking and reading about it, meant that moments after walking into the bookies, I was in my element.

The time was fast approaching 3 p.m. and Manchester United were kicking off in a matter of seconds. Unbeknown to me, in this place, that wasn't the event of paramount importance. That was the 'big' race about to start at Hamilton Park. I consulted the *Racing Post* that had been meticulously pinned to the corkboards around the shop, read the 'Verdict', and listened to two seasoned gamblers who had betting slips pouring out of their pockets or crumpled up in front of them. I coupled this research with instinct (I liked the name), and confidently wrote down my choice and circled it:

3.00pm @ Hamilton
£10
Majestic Roi
16/1

Between spins on the roulette wheel, I rushed over to place the bet then settled in for the race. I didn't hold out much hope for my horse or her jockey, Jamie Spencer, but who cared? I never expected to have even a tenner to play with when I woke up this morning.

As I learned was his style, Spencer would sit tight, leave it late and come from last to first to win by five lengths. BOOM – GET IN! As I clung to my betting slip, others around me were tearing up theirs or marching out of the shop – angry, annoyed and poorer. My football accumulator had already failed (no need to worry, there was always next time), so I thought I may as well see if the roulette wheel would remain kind before collecting my winnings from Hamilton Park. By the time Angie handed over £250 in fresh notes and I took my leave, I'd been in Coral for five hours.

That was easy and enjoyable, I thought to myself. I know loads about sport, and I can make loads of money while having loads of fun.

*   *   *

At this time, it's probably fair to say I wasn't any old teenager or first-year student: I was also a professional cricketer.

Aged 15, I'd been offered a place on the Academy of Northamptonshire CCC, one of English cricket's 18 first-class counties. Unlike many of my new teammates, I'd not previously played any junior county cricket, having been selected on the basis of my stellar performances at one of the country's top boarding schools, Oundle, where I'd been on a scholarship since the age of 13.

To be selected for the Academy was a dream come true, and preparation for a (hopefully long) career as a professional cricketer began. There were obvious but worthwhile sacrifices required for the remainder of my time at school as I played and trained with Northants, but this was all I'd ever wanted to do. Like so many others, I was desperate to make the game I loved into my job – and I was in a prime position to do so.

That dream moved a step closer when I left school and was offered a professional contract by Northants. The day I left school I moved to Northampton, where I lived in a house provided by the club on the edge of the county ground, Wantage Road, with four other professional cricketers. That summer, 2005, I was on an 'Emerging Player' contract, but was a full-time pro and played in the Second XI. In September, I signed a two-year deal.

This was undoubtedly brilliant and the opportunity of a lifetime. But as we left school, I experienced mixed emotions that I think act as a window into my personality. Mostly, this was because of 'FOMO' – Fear of Missing Out. It was one of my defining characteristics – I wanted to be involved with everything. Most of my mates were taking the well-trodden path of a gap year followed by university. They all had plans to jet off around the world, doing a ski season in the Alps, going to full moon parties in Thailand or saving the elephants through charity work in Africa. I was heading immediately into a rather more grown-up world and, while I knew what an opportunity awaited me, part of me wanted a slice of the fun they were about to experience.

But I also felt trepidation because I was stepping out of my comfort zone. I was going from being a very big fish in a small pond at school to being a nobody at the very bottom of a food chain, with everything to prove. At school I'd been high-achieving, popular, happy and totally comfortable in what I considered my perfect environment. Now I was entering the incredibly competitive and cut-throat world that I was so desperate to be a part of.

Originally the plan for my first winter as a pro, 2005–06, was to head to Australia (which would have helped ease my FOMO), but the club decided it was best for me to stay in Northampton, to get fit and try to add a yard of pace to my right-arm seamers. I had the fitness coach living with me and I trained hard, both with the county and at the National Performance Centre in Loughborough. There, I worked with Kevin Shine, the specialist fast-bowling coach, having impressed him when I played for England Schools earlier in the summer.

My first full summer, 2006, things went better than I – or indeed anyone else – expected. I started it by playing with the First XI in a pre-season friendly against Sussex at Hove, then spent the season playing for the county's Second XI with and against seasoned pros, including internationals. I enjoyed plenty of success, and my style of seam bowling was effective enough to put me on the verge of a debut for the first team in county cricket.

This was reflected when I received a call from Andy Moles, the former Warwickshire batsman and then England U19 Head Coach, asking me to come to Sleaford in Lincolnshire to play for an ECB Development of Excellence XI.

I arrived at the hotel in Sleaford not knowing what to expect but overcome with excitement (a giddy call to my dad on the journey reflected this), and was promptly told I would be playing against the touring India U19s the next day. Despite being bowled for a first-ball duck and having my bowling dispatched to all parts of the ground by none other than the now-legendary Virat Kohli, it was one of the proudest days of my life. I can take consolation from the fact that I wasn't the last bowler taken down by Kohli, who'll be remembered as one of the greatest batsmen of all time. Ishant Sharma, who has taken 300 Test wickets, was also in India's squad for that tour.

Despite boosting my pride, playing that game was a curse as well as a blessing. I had also been spending a lot of time around the Northants first team, often as 12th man, and both factors began to make me believe I'd made it, or at least that making it was inevitable. For the first time in my quest to reach the top of the game, complacency crept in.

And I had a decision to make. Throughout a summer that was going very well and giving me a welcome taste of life as a professional cricketer, a tricky choice was looming: to go to university, or not? In 2005, I'd deferred my place at Durham to study Combined Social Sciences in order to pursue professional cricket. The question now was whether to continue on that path, and throw myself into ensuring my Northants contract was extended at the end of the summer of 2007. An enjoyable winter playing in Australia was on the table, too.

Or I could go to university in Loughborough, my second choice. Loughborough was attractive because the cricket facilities and coaching were outstanding, and Northampton was just an hour away, close enough to pop back to train and play. Northants were certainly keen on this option.

After much deliberation I went, instead, for Durham. This way I could combine getting a degree from one of the best universities in the world with high-class cricket at the MCC Centre of Excellence (there were six of these at universities across the country, including at Durham) under the tutelage of Graeme 'Foxy' Fowler, the former England batsman. A number of top players, including England star Andrew Strauss, had taken this longer route into the game, which also provided the security of a good degree if things didn't go to plan in the unforgiving environment of professional sport. This looked a very sensible path indeed.

That Saturday in Coral came just a couple of weeks after my arrival in Durham and from that day onwards, I would find myself in a betting shop or casino at some point every single day. My successes on my first day as a gambler, and the feeling of true elation that brought me, immediately drew me back for more and more.

Finding the time wasn't hard: I had cricket commitments, but only 10 hours of lectures or seminars each week. I would nip in to the bookies before watching football with my mates in the pub, or do battle with the roulette table at Aspers casino after a night out. I could be in either for hours, and being just £10 down was cause for celebration.

The acceleration of my newfound hobby was exacerbated by my financial situation. It might seem strange to speak of having more money as a problem, but that was the situation I found myself in. I was different to most students as I had three income streams. My parents generously gave me an allowance (which was clearly, in hindsight, totally unnecessary), I had a sizeable student loan, and on top of that, Northants were paying me a salary to play cricket.

Money wasn't something that I thought about much, to be honest. I'd never been motivated by it. I didn't want the life of a professional cricketer for the fortune, I wanted it because I loved the game and competition. Growing up, I'd been frugal and spoke about saving (my family thought it entertaining how sensible I was with money). I had certainly not been one of those teenagers who spend every penny as soon as it lands with them. And in the world I inhabited, in the confines of boarding school and my full focus on becoming a professional cricketer, I'd not had much to spend money on anyway – until I arrived at Durham.

So as a student I was lucky that I didn't face the financial struggles that most students do. I didn't have to worry about whether it was either a late-night kebab or a trip to the sandwich shop for lunch the following day. I could afford to do both.

It also meant, though, that I was able to stick a few quid on both Lionel Messi to score a Champions League hat-trick and have a spin on the roulette wheel. Whereas I'd once been cautious with cash, now I had something that I really liked spending it on. And to me, the idea of watching a big game that I had a couple of quid on in the company of my mates and a few pints was absolute bliss.

And those Saturday trudges to Coral became the highlight of the week, easing a few more hangovers during the following months. The trip to Greggs beforehand became a ritual, and we would all take £20 of our student loans into the bookies.

I would sit at the roulette machine with mates at either shoulder instructing me which number to back next and going mad when a 20p stake came in. The aim of playing on the machine was to grow our pot to bet on the sports that between us we all shared a passion for – football, cricket and rugby. The improbability of many of the bets I was placing added to the enjoyment; if these 14 football teams that I know next to nothing about win, I'll turn a pound coin into half a million quid! Trust me, lads, there's a good chance of that happening.

We would bet on horses too, and loved scouring the *Racing Post*. We'd often all back the same horse in the hope that we could all celebrate together. And when we had money on all sorts of different sports, when one of us won (even just a few quid), it felt like we all won. If it didn't happen, it wasn't the end of the world. And so a combination of a lot of hope and very little expectation produced a lot of pleasure.

So more often than not, at the beginning, I would be gambling with other people – but I would do it alone too. I'd pop into the bookies if I had an hour or two between lectures and would be ecstatic if I made just five quid profit. It was my new thing, and I therefore wanted to do it a lot, as I'd always been an all-or-nothing character. I was a serial socialiser who loved being around people, and loved throwing myself into things.

Take sports training. Obviously, the fact that I loved playing and practising helped my cricket a lot, but I'd been obsessive about other sports, too. At school, I'd been a very solid rugby player, lining up in various positions in the backs. I wasn't the most talented goal-kicker around, but I enjoyed it a lot and saw what Jonny Wilkinson (this was around the time that he was in his pomp) achieved through obsessive dedication to improvement. So, I too practised religiously, desperate to become the best.

When I liked doing something, I tended to *really* like doing it. The same was true of my gambling, which was all great fun. It was something we generally did together as mates, providing hours of entertainment, spicing up the sport we would inevitably watch anyway, prompting some spontaneous nights out when things went well and, frankly, not much hardship when they didn't. At the time, it didn't appear to pose any problems at all.

What I found so satisfying about gambling, from my very first bet, was that it fulfilled my competitive needs. It allowed me to win or lose on tap. Obviously, I much preferred the winning, but it was the sense of it mattering, having a dog in the fight, that really got me going.

Being competitive was just part of me. Growing up, everything had been a competition or a challenge. My childhood was spent around the prep schools that my parents taught at, so there were always sports facilities available. My brother, younger by three years and owner of the same bright red hair, and I were constantly competing, between ourselves or with friends. If we went on holiday, there was no mucking about; we'd be tallying up points across different disciplines over the course of the week. I loved every minute of it. I thought winning, and being the best, was everything.

This did mean that, as a child, I was an awful loser. Aged 13 or 14, I would throw my toys out of the pram in toe-curling fashion when I lost or things didn't go to plan. There was one incident when Dad and I were playing in a fathers-and-sons golf competition. The format was foursomes, which means you play as a pair and take alternate shots. We were doing well but, on the final hole, my dad hit the ball into a bunker. These things happen and it was therefore my job to get us out of it. I failed to get us out of trouble, and completely lost my head – with my dad and the world more widely. I was apoplectic. It must have been very embarrassing for my dad.

I mellowed a little over the years – learning to manage my flame-haired instincts slightly better – but my competitive streak remained. I loved playing games and always felt they mattered. Gambling, my new hobby, struck a real sweet spot.

Despite gambling playing a role in my life that grew by the day, my first year at university passed without incident. Life was good and I was happy. My cricketing education was certainly more central to my life than its academic equivalent. Just like everyone else, I wasn't required to study much in order to get through first year and my focus lay elsewhere.

In April, our winter's work under Foxy Fowler was rewarded with first-class matches (this is what the 18 counties play, and is the highest level of cricket below the international game) against various counties, as traditional curtain-raisers for the new County Championship season. We faced Nottinghamshire, Lancashire and Durham, coming up against a host of internationals like Graeme Swann, David Hussey and Liam Plunkett. It was great fun, a great education and our team – which featured a number of guys who would go on to enjoy decent county careers – acquitted itself well. And for an inexperienced first-year student, I fared pretty well too, picking up a couple of four-wicket hauls.

In a flash, my fresher's year was over. I'd excelled at cricket and breezed through my exams. My liver had taken a hammering, I had a few relationship scars, and using those little blue biros in the bookies meant my bank balance wasn't as healthy as it might have been – but it had been a blast.

I left Durham in confident mood, hopeful that 2007 would be my breakthrough summer with Northants, which would lead to a contract extension before I headed back to the North East four months later.

3

June 2007

A few weeks after returning to Northampton, I spent some time out with an ankle injury. Injuries are an inevitable part of life as a professional sportsman but the way I'm wired meant that the first significant one I suffered wasn't easy for me to endure. I've never been someone who's good at just idling. I get bored easily and hate it, needing constant stimulation and to be on the go.

I was out for a month – hardly the end of the world – but I'd rarely, if ever, had nothing to do for that long, and I struggled. Time on a physio bed receiving treatment, or lying on a Swiss ball in the gym and swimming lengths alone in order to accelerate my rehabilitation was my idea of hell.

It was worsened by the knowledge that my teammates were out on the field doing what they loved, experiencing the buzz that only sport – especially at such a high level – can bring, before regaling everyone about it all in the bar afterwards. I missed that rush and, to make matters worse, newer, younger players were emerging at the club and around the country. I felt in stasis and in danger of being left behind.

I didn't like this, or know how to deal with it. I was only 20, but I was fiercely competitive and a little paranoid. I didn't know what to do with myself. So, the void I felt in my life was filled by indulging in my newest passion. In my time off, my day's rehabilitation work finished earlier than everyone else, so I could get to the bookies earlier and research the horses – something that a year earlier would have seemed totally barmy. I wasn't tired because I wasn't playing, so I would regularly go to the casino in the evening. I wasn't breaking any rules and I had the disposable income to fund my habit, but gambling was occupying my thoughts more and more.

I had only had a month off but already my lifestyle had changed. Soon enough, I was fit again and the problem wasn't that I wasn't playing, but that I was. I had to find the time for gambling, as well as doing a challenging job that I hadn't yet cracked.

When once I had considered myself the hardest-working player – first into training, last out – that quickly changed. The thought of staying late to run a few miles on the treadmill, bowling or hitting a few more balls, or working with a senior player on my technique was suddenly being replaced by a need to head to the local Ladbrokes to have a punt on the afternoon's racing.

Gambling was soon demanding my time, money and thoughts. I would walk into the bookies with a £20 note when the 1.10 at Catterick was about to start, and I would walk out as England's cricketers left the field for bad light shortly before 7 p.m. One of the many issues with this was that, while I would walk out with £250 in my hand, I would have conveniently erased from my memory that I'd actually been to the cashpoint several times while in the shop.

My cricket couldn't keep up with this. Frankly I wasn't talented enough to not give absolutely every ounce of myself, and I was slowly found out. It was the latter half of the summer and that wasn't good news for me either; as a seamer, my bowling style meant I was a real force in the early months of the summer when my lack of pace didn't matter too much. As the sunshine arrived and the wickets became better for batting,

I needed to bring my A-game every single day. Needless to say, I wasn't doing that.

And then there was the socialising. The world of Second XI county cricket is a very strange environment. It's the meeting of many different types of cricketer. Like me, there are youngsters trying to make their way in the game, chasing a place in the first team. On their way up in the world, they're generally ambitious and professional. Then there are first team players, sometimes big names, who've been dropped or are returning from injury. They don't have to work too hard to succeed at this level. Alongside them there are triallists who have come from club cricket or have been released by other counties. No one really wants them to do well, as they're a threat from outside.

And then there are the guys who rip it up in the Seconds but struggle when asked to take the step up to the first team. In my time at Northants, this group were big characters who were a fair bit older than me. They would go out drinking on away trips and still have no problem doing their job adequately the following day.

I thought I could do the same but it wasn't that easy. I was young, insecure, impressionable and desperate to be liked and accepted. I got on with these guys, and started to tag along with some of the less professional aspects of their lifestyle because I was never strong enough to say 'no'. I was no good at sitting around in a hotel room; I needed to be doing something, rather than resting and relaxing. So, I would get drunk with them, or I would go gambling alone. As you can imagine, neither was good for my cricket.

As a team, we generally struggled. Other counties had more money and deeper squads, so we often knew we weren't going to win the game a day or two from its end. Needless to say, that only encouraged us to have some fun. Without really noticing, I'd rather lost my way.

The end of August, with the season approaching its end, is cricket's contract season and a nervy time for those whose deals are up – the situation I found myself in in 2007. At this time, players and their agents meet coaches and club chief executives to thrash out deals, and dressing rooms are quieter and emptying. Northants had been through some challenging times on and off the field, and all of us who were out of contract knew anything was possible.

I had the awareness to realise that I'd not had a great year, but I was only 20 and still at university, so wouldn't cost as much to keep as a full-time or more experienced player. There was still a chance I would be kept on. Deep down, though, I knew it was really a question of whether the club believed in my ability to really crack the top level in the long term. I now understand why the answer was 'no', and when I look back, I sense my teammates probably knew that, and so did my parents and mates away from the game. Of course, at the time I was confident in my own abilities.

Moments before going into my meeting, on 1 September, 2007, I was told that Usman Afzaal – a Test cricketer who had played in the Ashes six years earlier – had been informed that he was being released by the club. Suddenly, I was overcome with fear.

But I still wasn't prepared to hear, in the Chief Executive's office, that my contract was also not being renewed. Just like that, my dream was shattered. I took the news on the chin but it hit me very hard, and I was hurting. I had never been told by anyone that I wasn't good enough – especially not at cricket, which had always been my thing.

I had no experience of dealing with rejection, or lived through any personal crisis, and therefore no training for this situation or how I would react to it. My coping mechanism was to act how I thought you were supposed to in such situations: to 'man up' and show no vulnerability – even if vulnerable was exactly how I was feeling.

I had always feared failure but had little experience of it. My life had been going to plan and I'd always succeeded at everything I tried. I was a perfectionist who had been a high achiever coming through school and had spent that first year at uni having my ego pumped up more. Now, my bubble had been well and truly burst.

The process of leaving the club was brutal. With the Second XI games done for the season, so was my time at the club – with immediate effect. I walked out of the office, processing some of the worst news I'd ever received, and walked upstairs to the changing rooms to pack up my kit. The first team were playing a County Championship game at home so there were several lads about. I said goodbye to them, the physio who had helped me earlier that summer, and some of the other support staff.

I was still living in a house next to the cricket ground, so went straight up there and packed my stuff up. That night, I went to the pub with a few of the players who lived locally, but I never got to say goodbye to some of the other lads. The next morning, I drove out of the ground and that was that. I heard nothing more from the club, received no support, and didn't return for more than five years. The Professional Cricketers' Association (PCA) dinner, the players' big end-of-season knees-up in London, was taking place a few weeks later and I'd planned to go. But having just been released, I couldn't face it.

Instead, having received my final month's salary for September, I flew to Morocco two days later with my girlfriend. My parents were in the process of moving from Derbyshire to Sussex to continue their teaching careers, so I didn't even have anywhere particularly familiar to go to.

I found telling people – friends, family and teammates – that I'd been released extremely hard, all linked to that fear of failure. I'd always been good at telling people good news but tended to keep bad news to myself. I remember calling my dad and being gripped by fear that he would be hugely disappointed in me. Of course, he was incredibly supportive and very relaxed. I rang Foxy Fowler, who expressed shock, surprise and even anger because he was a coach who would always back his players to the hilt. But generally, I waited for people to ask rather than just telling them straight up and owning it.

Becoming a professional cricketer – not just someone who played the game, but someone who would earn a living for many years doing it – had been central to my identity throughout my teens, even before I got a contract. When I went back to Durham the following month, I found life much more difficult. In my first year, my contract, being a pro and being paid had made me a bit of a big deal. I hated that this was no longer the case. Freshers joined the cricket club over the following two years with county contracts, but I'd lost mine.

People liked talking to me about my professional career, I loved telling them about it and it swelled my ego. Now that career looked doubtful to those on the outside, and dead in the water to me. Put simply, I was embarrassed and felt like I'd let people down. It didn't help that many of my teammates seemed to think I was very hard done by. It was nice to hear them say I should have been kept on but it didn't change anything and only added to that bitterness.

I started questioning lots of what I'd done. Should I have gone to Loughborough University, not Durham, as Northants had wanted? Should I have bothered going to university at all? Would everything have been different if they had encouraged me to go to Australia that winter?

Even if I lacked a bit of pace, I was a very good bowler when conditions suited me, but my batting left me harbouring regrets. I had talent with the bat, but had never scored the volume of runs to back that up. I should have been competing for that most competitive spot in the cricket team – the genuine all-rounder – but my batting held me back. I'd found school cricket simple, taking lots of wickets and scoring runs down the batting order, but that probably didn't serve me well when making the vast step up to county and first-class level.

There was an element of resentment, too. I knew I wasn't as good as some of those around me and Northants were telling me I wasn't good enough to make it by releasing me. But had I really ever had the chance to prove that I was good enough to make it? I'd come very close to the first team but never actually been given a shot, despite strong performances for the second team and in first-class cricket for the university. I just wanted a chance to show them they were wrong. The club employed lots of experienced, top-class South African players at the time, which made opportunities harder to come by for young, local players like me. For a few years, I had mixed emotions watching some of my contemporaries enjoy success in the game.

So I questioned a lot of things – but not the fact that I'd screwed up. I'd spent so much time gambling lately that I'd taken my eye off the ball. I was only 20, but being released by Northants left me feeling like my cricket career was over and that there was no way back. Playing cricket professionally was all I'd ever really thought about doing, initially at least. Having fallen out of the system, getting back in would be mighty tough.

Foxy was convinced that I would be picked up by another county at some stage, and I continued to perform pretty solidly for the university. But I now had considerable self-doubt and didn't think I could make it. I looked back on things that had happened that summer and convinced myself that they were proof that I wasn't good enough. At the time, they had just seemed like little bumps in the road. Now, they seemed like evidence that the whole road was blocked.

For example, when I came back from my ankle injury, I played for the Seconds against our Warwickshire counterparts. We batted first and declared six wickets down, so I didn't get a bat. When we took the field, we had a strong attack so I was the sixth bowler used, not coming on until after the 30th over, which didn't play to my strengths at all. When I finally came on, Vaughn van Jaarsveld – who would go on to play a few internationals for South Africa – was in. My first three balls to him, which were all perfectly good deliveries, were launched for three of the biggest sixes I have seen. After the third I just laughed and said to him, 'What have I done to deserve this?' His reply didn't mess about: 'Mate, I was watching you in the warm-up and have been waiting for you to come on to bowl.'

Earlier that year, playing for the university in a first-class game against a strong Lancashire side, I'd experienced another hammering. It had been a good game, and Lancashire were chasing about 260 to win in the fourth innings. We reduced them to 56 for five, so had a sniff, and I bowled a pretty decent first spell. Then Steven Mullaney, who was a similar age to me and has gone on to be a superb county cricketer, got going. He made 165 not out to win the game, including smacking the first over of my second spell for five sixes. Ouch.

Being released didn't mean that there would be no more opportunities in the game, but that wasn't my reading of the situation. I felt done. I continued playing, but held no hope that it would give me the career I craved. I had two more years at Durham, which meant three more first-class games each spring, and in 2008 I went on to tour Cape Town with British Universities, then spent two months on trial with Kent, playing for the Second XI.

But while I was a student, I was able to put off the thought of exactly what came next. I didn't yet need another career.

Meanwhile, in October 2007, I returned to Durham for my second year, having enjoyed my holiday in Morocco, without my county contract and with considerably less drive – even if that wasn't obvious to those around me.

Uni was different this year as I'd moved out of the gloomy cell in Hild-Bede College and into a house with six mates. I had a double bed, we had a bar in the living room and endless other means of entertainment to distract us from our studies over the next nine months.

I had an even better distraction, though. Slowly but surely, I was unwittingly getting more and more into gambling. At that time, it felt the perfect drug for me: it was fun; it involved sport; it didn't eat up time that was valuable; I could do it, and talk about it, with my mates (it wasn't *all* we talked about…); I could afford it; it didn't majorly impact my studies, which I continued to pass seamlessly; and it was the closest thing I could find to replicate the buzz of playing cricket, the thing I loved most as a competitive beast.

Cricket had given me such a rush – the acts of taking a wicket or hitting a boundary, but also the camaraderie in a team, playing in front of crowds, and people wanting to talk to you about the game. The only thing I could find that came close was gambling. It gave me instant gratification – whether I won or lost. It gave me that buzz, and also allowed me an escape from the problems I felt but was hiding from others.

Gambling wasn't teaching me any tough lessons, either. There were bad weeks, where I'd suffer some briefly alarming losses of about £250. But the stakes were low enough that there were just as many good weeks where I'd win big. Me and my mates would still indulge in our Saturday fun, but I would pop in alone between lectures – with increasing frequency. And then, when I intended to squeeze 30 minutes of guilt-free gambling into my day, it would turn into a couple of hours, which meant missing lectures. It wasn't rare for me to go to the bookies more than once a day, and I started going to more obscure gambling shops that my mates were less likely to be in.

I began to enjoy gambling alone a bit more, because it allowed me to be more aggressive in my approach – higher stakes and more bets. This was perhaps a subconscious acknowledgement that I was doing something wrong or naughty. As I was obsessed with being successful, and those around me considering me successful (or, put another way, so fearful of failure and those around me considering me a failure), I'd hidden things over the years. God forbid that my parents would catch wind that I liked smoking from time to time. I also recognised that gambling in the volumes that I was racking up was bad and that there was a stigma around it. I didn't want to be judged.

It was also 'me time'. On one such occasion I'd driven to a branch of William Hill in Durham that wasn't often frequented by students. It was near a massive supermarket, though, so there was at least an excuse to be in the area. I was 'doing a weekly shop'. I'd been in there for some time, playing on the roulette machine. I'd managed to rack up a very significant pot of about £500, which was unusually large at a time when I saw £100 as a big win.

I'd developed theories about the machines, and which numbers followed which. For example, when 11, 22 or 33 came up, another of those numbers would follow immediately after. On this occasion I'd plenty of cash to play with so thought I'd test my theory. The maximum you could stake on a number was £13, which would result in a win of £500. Twenty-two appeared, so I backed 11 and 33 with the full £13, put a bit on 22 again and a little on green zero too – because nothing annoyed me more than that coming up when I hadn't backed it. My little theory came good: the virtual ball bearing dropped into the 33 slot, and I suddenly had close to £1,000 in the bank!

Almost simultaneously, one of my best mates walked into the shop. What are the chances? He also loved a flutter and, like me, bet a bit more than he let on to everyone else. We had made no plans to meet so there was a little awkwardness as our eyes met but we were there for the same reason and didn't need to say anything to confirm that our secret was mutually safe.

And then he walked over, saw my screen and was immediately taken aback. He insisted that I withdrew the money immediately – which I did. I don't know whether I would have had the self-control to withdraw the money had he not walked in. So we left together and I'd won money I could only dream of, some of which went on an extremely fun night out. We didn't mention our meeting to anyone else but it wasn't the last time we would bump into one another in that same shop in Framwellgate.

By now, I wasn't just taking £20 in to a shop like I once had, I was arriving with my wallet and wasn't afraid of going back and forth from the ATM. For the first time, I started chasing losses. If £10 went into the machine, £10 had to come out; £2 on a roulette spin became £5 a time; and 20p on my favourite numbers became 80p. The £1 pipedream accumulators to become a student millionaire became £10 strategic six-fold multi-bets that I expected to happen, and when they didn't my reaction was anger, rather than disappointment. When I placed 'the same' bets as my mates, as we had started doing in our first year, I would now have a higher stake that they didn't know about. So, it mattered that bit more. When they lost those bets, they were irritated. When I lost those bets, I was furious.

I became more and more interested in horse racing, attempting to study form and monitoring the activity of the handicapper. My mates noticed this and used me as an amateur tipster and source of knowledge. My ego, dented by the cricket disappointment, swelled. Losing didn't ruin my day, but it did influence it. At this time, I viewed gambling almost entirely through a financial prism: wins and losses. But it also played a part in personal trials and tribulations. It could no longer just be contained as a quiet thing I did on my own.

I was lying a lot to those important to me, including my girlfriend. We had met in freshers' week and had been together for two years. She was brilliant. She knew nothing of the extent of my gambling because it was a dirty secret that I was keeping from everyone. Lying about it – where I'd been, what I was up to – became increasingly natural, compulsive, even. And that lying was contagious, so I became increasingly dishonest about other topics.

And so, at the start of my third year at Durham, that long-term relationship broke down in hugely dishonest and regrettable fashion on my part. Let's just say that you can't help who you fall for, but falling for the girlfriend of your former housemate when you are already in a (terrific) relationship is clearly a recipe for disaster.

This situation – which ended with me in a new relationship – showed that I'd become untrustworthy, that I was someone who thought they could have it all, and always wanted more. I couldn't just settle for my already-amazing lot and got bored easily. I lacked self-control, had little regard for anyone but myself and didn't think about consequences before I acted. My new girlfriend was considered cool and a great catch. I liked that people knew I was going out with her.

So I was lying a lot and had become rather erratic. But the only visible scars of that were that I'd lost a couple of friends in the break-up. On the surface of things, I remained a high-achieving young bloke with plenty going for him.

I was still able to spend the best part of two years captaining the university cricket team, which is something I'm incredibly proud of. I played alongside future internationals and T20 guns for hire, as well as some of the country's best county and club cricketers. We made some great memories and had a brilliant time playing under Foxy.

By my third year at uni, Fox was calling me Benjamin Button, after the fictional character who ages in reverse. I'd arrived as this hard-working, driven, sensible, grown-up professional and was leaving as a loose character who had regressed. It was all tongue in cheek, and Foxy didn't suspect the real reason this was happening, but he was a sharp judge of character and was certainly on to something.

So the summer of 2009 arrived, I got the 2:1 degree result I wanted without too much hassle, and it was time to fully admit that a career as a professional cricketer wasn't going to happen.

What next? Do I follow my parents into teaching? Follow my mates into the rat race of the city? Try to make my passion for sport work somehow in my life? Unlike many of my peers I'd not been on summer internships each year because I'd been playing cricket.

I chose to keep my options open and gain experience in different areas. The big decisions could wait. First, that meant playing some club cricket with mates, getting my golf handicap down and clinging onto a student lifestyle.

Then came a brief internship with a small sports agency in London, which seemed an appealing path. They provided me with a great opportunity but it served to reveal how tough a career it would be without a long career in sport behind me, with the status and contacts that would bring. It was also not quite as glamorous as I thought and, in fact, involved menial administrative tasks like booking flights and ordering trainers.

Why not try teaching? As both of my parents were teachers, I was familiar with this world and also aware of its many benefits – the long holidays and nice lifestyle. I knew rather better what I was getting myself into, especially as the school I was going to gain experience at was run by my father. For the autumn term of 2009 I worked on the Sussex Downs, teaching PE and coaching sport while living with my parents. This had the added benefit of allowing me to save some money for whatever I wanted to try next and, as much as I enjoyed experiencing a rewarding (and exhausting) profession, there was a nagging feeling that I still really wanted to try out big business in the bright lights of London.

I applied for various graduate schemes and finally got lucky after another personal connection came good. The CEO of an international insurance broker also happened to be the MCC Universities mentor at Durham and, after a long chat, I was offered an interview for a graduate position at the company. I knew next to nothing about insurance – other than that it was something you got for your car or before you went on holiday in case you got into a scrape while drunk – but I navigated my way through the interview and was offered the job later in the day.

Those months since university had only moved my gambling forwards. I would still go to the betting shop every day, gambling on almost all sporting events and spending any spare time playing on the fixed odds machines. I was betting heavily on golf, and spent a lot of time looking into horses in search of tips. I even went to race meets regularly when I could in the evening. I'd no debts, but no savings either, and everything I'd earned in cricket was gone.

My parents were, by now, aware that I gambled – mainly because of one major lapse of judgement earlier in the year. With my parents busy at school, I offered to do the weekly shop for them. It was a helpful act that doubled as a front for me to nip into the bookies for 20 minutes while in town. With my funds low – not unusual, they thought, for someone who had just returned from university – Mum lent me her debit card and told me the PIN. Having ticked off every item on the long shopping list with ruthless precision, I headed for a quick spin on the roulette machine.

'Quick' ended up meaning more than four hours, the emptying of my (shallow) account, and the withdrawal of the maximum daily allowance on hers. As if nothing had happened, I returned home and unloaded the shopping (some of which could probably have done with being in the fridge for a couple of hours). I left the receipt very visibly on the side.

At the time, bank statements were a monthly business. And my mum checked hers carefully. When it arrived some weeks later, I couldn't hide. I came clean, but put my error down to a moment of madness induced by boredom and poverty. They were angry and disappointed, and I received a major dressing down. I paid them back as soon as I could. As time passed, little more was said about it. My explanations were accepted and my naivety blamed.

Before heading off to join most of Durham University's graduates in south-west London to try to earn our fortunes, I enjoyed a lovely family Christmas at home. Little did I know, I was entering an environment that would act as a catalyst for my secret addiction.

4

January 2010

There was so much in London that was new to me. I'd never lived in a big city and never had a proper office job. It's barely an exaggeration to say that every single thing I was doing at this time was unwittingly playing into the hands of my developing addiction.

I'd decided to move in with three of my closest mates from Durham but, while we searched for a house, I flitted between my girlfriend's mother's house and some generous family friends' place, as I had done while doing the sports agency internship a few months earlier.

It was a couple of months before we found 44a Lambrook Terrace, just off Fulham Palace Road, and it was just what we were after. It was a short walk from our favourite pubs, a stone's throw from a Tesco Express, and close to various stations for our different commutes. We soon learned that we lived on the same street as The Saturdays' heartthrob Mollie King, which shows that these were plush surroundings for four 23-year-old graduates.

At about the same time, my girlfriend dumped me. She'd been thinking about going travelling for a while, but now definitely decided that she was off to Thailand with her best mate. In this plan, there was no space for a boyfriend back home (despite my protestations), as it would merely cramp her style. I'd burned a few bridges to get this relationship off the ground and I was in denial that it was over. She clearly wasn't so bothered; I learned pretty promptly from Facebook that she was enjoying a holiday romance.

Being dumped by my girlfriend, like being dumped by Northants, was a dent to my ego. I'd always felt that I was punching above my weight – besides the fact that I loved her, it was a relationship I loved being part of. Less than 18 months earlier, I'd lost some friends permanently for this. All dumpings hurt but this one felt costly, too. I went into tailspin. I couldn't see any viable alternative to life with her.

I tried to talk to my parents about how I was feeling but I just couldn't admit how much it was affecting me, or ask for help. My approach was to run away from the problem – and go to my safe space: watching a roulette wheel spin, watching a horse run, or drinking lager at pace. All those around me could see I was in pieces but I used gambling to convince myself that all was well, and used the break-up as an excuse to gamble. And naturally, I gambled more and more.

It was escapism. I wanted to avoid thinking about what was going on. As soon as I stopped gambling, I would think about my broken heart again. In the past, my excesses had been a way of combatting boredom, but right now they were a way of combatting a traumatic event. That escapism is, in its own way, pretty addictive. This, then, was a tumultuous time to be settling into a new job in a new city.

Insurance is an extraordinary industry that is not easy to explain to the uninitiated. In my experience, it was built on interpersonal relationships and mixing socialising with business. I wasn't expected to sit at a computer firing off emails or making calls all day. Instead, every day in the middle of the morning I would wander 15 minutes from the office to Lloyd's of London, a huge building that had lifts that looked like tins of canned soup on its exterior, then run around this unusual 'market place' getting contracts signed. I'd be there from about

11 a.m. until 1 p.m., at which point Lloyd's would close for an hour and a half.

Then followed a long and usually boozy lunch. Once that was done I had a decision to make: return to the office to write a few fuzzy emails and make some calls, or head back to Lloyd's (which was open again from about 2.30 until 4 p.m.) to have a few more informal chats with the resident underwriters (this counted as 'work'), or even have a few more pints until we drew stumps – sometimes deep into the evening. The first option was the most sensible, the second was a token gesture. There are no prizes for guessing which was the most common course of action.

As my movements and time weren't managed closely, I added a few extra layers to my working day. On my morning walk from the office to Lloyd's I would visit at least one of the numerous bookies en route for a few spins of roulette or a bit of blackjack.

And lunch would usually be preceded by a trip to one of the numerous bookies just outside Lloyd's. I would regularly head through the doors, down the stairs and into a gambler's paradise. The purpose of this trip was always to get in there before the afternoon horse racing started so that when I returned after lunch I would either have won a tidy sum or have to work doubly hard in the afternoon session. If for whatever reason lunch rumbled on, then there would inevitably be an early evening visit, with me now under the influence and feeling a little more courageous.

On the post-lunch trip particularly, it wasn't uncommon to be in the company of many others I knew from the insurance circuit. Bosses would think we were back in Lloyd's working but instead we'd be having a punt after an extremely efficient morning session at Lloyd's. That was increasingly how I approached my day – to absolutely cram like a maniac in the morning so that my afternoon was free for a trip to the bookies, the pub or both. I could walk back into the office at 4 p.m. and it looked like I'd been at Lloyd's all day.

It helped that gambling was part of the insurance culture. People would talk about horse racing or football odds in the pub. We'd gossip about senior management owning horses or having a box at Aintree or Ascot. Stepping into such an environment when I was grieving for my relationship and wanted distraction accelerated my gambling rapidly.

As the weekend approached, I would socialise heavily with my mates, either with pints in Parson's Green pubs or going out to the clubs on the King's Road. Either way, I would almost inevitably eventually find myself in the Grosvenor Casino at Gloucester Road.

For the first time in my life, I wasn't bound to an institution. I'd been to junior schools where my dad was the headmaster, then to boarding school until I was 18. From there, I spent a year under the close watch of Northants before going to university, where I spent the next three years.

There are not only rules to follow, but pressures attached to being at those institutions. And I put my own pressure on myself because I was desperate to be seen as this high-achiever in those environments, where every success is measured. That pressure weighed on me. I thought it was the be-all and end-all to achieve in the accepted manner.

But now, turning 24, I felt I had done pretty well so far, had a good job and was my own man. My work required some respect, but I wasn't there 24/7 like at school or university. For much of the time I could do what I wanted.

And, in short, I chose to party and gamble. Exacerbated by the break-up, I was burning the candle at both ends with at least one of my housemates several nights a week. In truth, most of my mates were riding a similar wave, living a wild existence drinking and gambling with the occasional one night stand thrown in.

There were plenty of days when I'd go out for lunch, get hammered, have one of my afternoons in the betting shop, then off to the pub, the casino and home to bed. I'd fall asleep in my suit, wake up to my fifth and final alarm and leg it straight to the office wearing the same clothes. Then do it all again. Plenty of people turned up to work hungover, but few took as many Friday sickies as I did. I was lucky not to be pulled up on it.

When I made those trips to the casino, I was gambling just as aggressively and excessively as I was in the daytime around work, just in a different environment. I remember, on a number of occasions, going to the casino cashpoint (the sort that charges you £2.75 for a withdrawal) at 11.59 p.m. and taking out my daily limit of £250, then returning a couple of minutes later when the clock had passed midnight to make exactly the same withdrawal.

Somehow, through all this, I appeared to be quite good at my job. Broking came quite naturally to me and I was learning fast about the ins and outs of the world of public liability insurance. When I needed to be, I was the consummate professional and appeared to those above and around me to be taking to this industry like a duck to water.

But the truth was that I was winging it, basing it all on personality and charm, and my behaviour in my personal life was very immature. I was being allowed to make decisions for myself for the first time ever and was fully taking advantage of that. Looking back , it's actually frightening to think that I was handling million-pound insurance deals while half-cut.

By December, almost a year in, I was summoned to a meeting with the CEO, as my graduate contract was coming to an end. It was an intimidating environment, with the Head of UK Operations, the Head of Liability Division (my boss) and the Head of HR – who was known by some in the office as the 'Grim Reaper' as she seemed to come down from another branch exclusively to give bad news – all present.

I need not have worried, as I was showered with praise and given a lavish promotion, pay rise and Christmas bonus. I couldn't shake their hands and get out of the door quickly enough – this was great news, for both my professional and private lives.

Like many competitive, ego-driven young males, I didn't like keeping good news to myself for long, just as I didn't like telling a soul when I had bad news. Just as I'd been desperate to hide that I'd been released by Northants, I now had to let my mates know immediately about my promotion, and promised that I would be getting the drinks in the following evening, Wednesday, with my newfound wealth. I was buzzing.

I started with a few pints at the Lamb at Leadenhall Market – a favourite spot on the insurance scene – then went to meet my uni mates at the APT bar, just around the corner from Bank station in the heart of the City, with St Paul's Cathedral in sight. This place suited us down to the ground, not least because it did buy-one-get-one-free pints 6–8 p.m. on Wednesdays and Thursdays.

And, conveniently for me, there was a tiny, often quiet William Hill two doors down that I could slip into before arriving or while pretending to have a Marlboro Light outside.

Much of my gambling was secretive – a long way from just being fun with mates.

I arrived 15 minutes earlier than I'd arranged to meet my friends, allowing me to stick some money on the Champions League games that were due to kick-off shortly. I felt emboldened by my bonus and the knowledge that – like my three income streams at university – this was money that I didn't necessarily need right now, especially with a pay rise round the corner. A bit of luck tonight and all my family would be getting lovely Christmas presents in a couple of weeks. I was also operating with a little extra confidence thanks to the pints I'd tucked into since work.

Dutch courage or not, my relationship with money was fast changing in London. Where once I'd been unmoved by it, my exposure to the wealth around me – in the office, on the streets – meant I wanted that, too. I wanted to be as successful as those working above me. I didn't mind my job but saw it as a means to an end, getting rich, earning bonuses and living a lavish lifestyle. If any of those around me working in the City denied that was their motivation, I reckon they were lying.

I'd spent the walk from the Lamb weighing up who I would back, and ramping up the stakes in my mind. I settled on a big accumulator – much bigger than ever before – and a number of smaller bets in case I was let down early. The accumulator included all six of the evening's Champions League games, and a web of possibilities; the odds were just shy of 70/1 and the stake. . . £500.

As I handed over the betting slip and my debit card, the lad behind the glass appeared shocked. I walked upstairs to meet my mates – who were blissfully unaware of what I'd been up to – and proceeded to get very drunk with them. A couple of hours later, all six results had gone my way. Over the course of just one evening, £500 had become £34,977.61.

Wow.

I was doing somersaults inside but I didn't tell a soul. I just settled the bar bill and left a hefty tip. I tried to make it appear as if nothing had changed. Rather a lot had changed, though. My muted reaction told the tale of my developing addiction, but I also now had my hands on a life-changing amount of money, more than most people earn in a year, a deposit for a dream home, or all sorts of other treats. I had all this and I was just 24.

My commitments – to drinking that evening and working the following morning – meant I wasn't able to return to collect my winnings until lunchtime on Thursday. This was such a large amount of money that the cashier at William Hill appeared to be waiting for me to arrive, and then – because the win was so big – was only able to give me the first £1,000 in cash. The rest could be deposited onto the card I paid with (which would take up to a week), paid by cheque, or given via a third option: placing the money in a William Hill online account.

I already had a couple of accounts with bookmakers but rarely used them. But this now seemed a viable option. I opted for a hybrid approach: £1,000 in cash, £5,000 back into my current account and the remaining £29,000 or so into my new online gambling account. In the time it took to administer these transactions, I managed to lose about £100 on the roulette machine, but I headed back to the office with a spring in my step, delighted with how my life had changed in the last 48 hours.

This was also such a large amount of money that it instantly changed me, as well as deepening my troubled approach to gambling. That win gave me a sort of hero complex, and I used the money to go out even more and to behave in ways I never had before.

I agreed to go on lavish holidays and trips. One, in March, was a tour to Hong Kong and China with the MCC (Marylebone Cricket Club), cricket's most iconic club and the custodians of Lord's, under the management of former England captain, Mike Gatting. I was extremely lucky to be invited – proper once-in-a-lifetime stuff.

I didn't treat it that way at all. Sure, I made the most of it, but I was out of control. I carried on like a millionaire. We drank very heavily, and my approach was to play hard, on and off the field. One morning, I missed the bus, having got in very late from a boozy one, and got a major telling-off from Gatting. He told me in no uncertain terms that if I stepped out of line again, I'd be sent home.

And then there was the inevitable gambling. It was illegal to gamble in Hong Kong, so me and a couple of others crossed the Pearl River Delta to Macau, in China. When there, we did all-nighters in the casino.

We also went to the iconic night racing at Happy Valley. All of us were putting on bets at the kiosks, but I was also placing huge bets online through Betfair. I'd no idea what I was doing but one of the other lads knew a bit about racing in Hong Kong and was advising me. My stakes were massive and I lost a lot of money.

That same month, I went on a lads' skiing holiday to Chamonix, in France. One day we woke up hungover and the conditions were absolutely horrendous, so we decided to have a day off skiing. We went for a big, boozy lunch before deciding to pop into a casino. As it was mid-afternoon, all the blackjack and roulette tables were shut, and only the slot machines were open. Most of the lads headed straight for the bar but me and one other stayed on for a flutter. I was playing the game 'higher or lower', in French. The machine would show a playing card, and my job was to guess whether the next one to be shown would be higher or lower. Without knowing what I was doing, I eventually won the jackpot – €2,500. My mate called the others, who came straight back in disbelief. Keen to make my mates think this was an extraordinary moment, and not the sort of money I won fairly often, I showered them with drinks and spent the whole lot that night.

Back home in London, I was going out all the time, and buying huge rounds of drinks and visiting strip clubs. I was smoking a lot more and even dabbling in Class A drugs, such as cocaine. I would never cook, just ordering takeaways and eating out.

I didn't think about saving any of this money. My big win made me believe that another one would be just around the corner, and also made me think that my stakes could rise. Ten pounds each way on a horse became £100. A £20 spin on the roulette wheel became £200.

Some of the raising of my stakes was down to knowledge. I was spending all my spare time scouring tipping websites and following those in the know about racing on social media. With this knowledge came confidence that I was going to win. Clearly that wasn't always the case. When I did win in the daytime, I was often emboldened to go to the casino in the evening. When I lost all my money there, I wouldn't be upset, thinking myself 'even' for the day.

Worst of all was that my huge Champions League win gave me a buzz that I could only replicate by bettering it. I would win £500, or even £1,000, on a horse, but it wasn't £35,000. Gambling was now something I wanted to do all the time.

Online gambling meant that I could, indeed, do it all the time. That I had 29 grand just sitting around in my account meant that my funds felt almost unlimited. It didn't feel like real money that I handed over to a cashier, or placed in a machine myself. This felt like Monopoly money. Pick who to back, and click. Win or lose. Simple.

Alongside being dumped and settling into a new place and job, there had been a third significant change to my life when I moved to London that didn't help my gambling either – it was the first time I had a smartphone. In fact, I had two. Work gave me a BlackBerry, which was strictly for business. And my personal phone was an iPhone, on which I had increasing numbers of apps, which opened up a whole new way of accessing gambling. The two different phones allowed me to keep some separation between work and play too – I never did any gambling on my BlackBerry. On the iPhone, I was always busy gambling away – it was so easy.

Gambling in shops, as I'd started out doing, was naturally a more controlled environment. You had the opportunity to simply walk out of the shop or casino, and there would come a point on every visit when you would have to. You would also have to load the machine or go to the cashier to make a bet, then return to the cashpoint – a moment of vague reflection – when you ran out of cash. Online betting, particularly on my phone, felt like a constant flow of chips rather than actual money that belonged to me. Whereas I'd once put money into machines £20 by £20, now I was betting £200 by £200. There's no difference in the amount you can bet in a shop or online, but using digital – not physical – currency meant the money flowed faster. When I walked into a bookmakers, I was limited by how much cash I had in my wallet. When I bet online, I was only limited by how much cash I had in my account.

I very rarely withdrew from my online accounts and if I did, it would be because I needed to pay for something urgently. Wins would stay in the account to fund the next bet, and when I lost, I would want to win it back quickly.

The upshot was that by the end of January 2011, six short weeks after my big win, my winnings were all gone, mainly on punts and pints. There were three significant issues here. One, I was desperate to win it back fast, and the inevitable method for achieving this was gambling. Two, the experience of winning really big meant I thought winning really big again was bound to happen. And three, I suddenly had a new standard of living to uphold. All three would rapidly change my life – financially, mentally and professionally – in the six months that followed.

I started to structure my day based on the sporting calendar, particularly racing, which happened in the afternoon. My trips to the bookies got longer and longer. My holidays would centre on Ebor – a racing festival in York in August – and Cheltenham, very different experiences to the family holidays I loved so much. One year at Cheltenham, a mate and I literally gambled everything we had, to the point where we had to borrow money from another friend's dad in order to get back to London and buy something to eat. In the summer of 2010, I had got quite into going out to the Windsor races on my own on a Monday evening. I would tell people it was a work trip, but I would just go and indulge in hours of gambling in isolation. By the summer of 2011, six months after my big win, I was doing this most weeks.

The guilt I felt about my gambling, which I'd first experienced in a small way at university, grew and grew. I really had something to hide now. I tried to remain motivated at work because, in an incentivised industry like insurance broking, better performance meant more money. More money meant more gambling.

But working in insurance, with all those bookies nearby and online accounts on your phone, gave me plenty of opportunities to gamble and there were signs that my focus wasn't actually on my job, as much as I might be leading myself and others to believe.

Gambling losses would badly affect my mood. I was often late for meetings and commitments. If I'd had a bad evening in the casino, I'd be reluctant to go into work the following day, pulling a sickie instead. I struggled for motivation after lunch if I'd endured a poor morning betting; my mind would automatically be elsewhere.

Often, it would be as simple as saying I was working when I was actually in the bookies. Instead of walking to Lloyd's at 11 a.m. as I should have done, I would head to a betting shop. I started putting fake lunch meetings in my diary so that others were none the wiser.

Away from work, I was becoming a master of disguise. Socially, I remained the life and soul of the party, game for anything at any time. I said yes to everything. This was an important image for me to maintain as it revealed no chinks in my armour. My friends knew I gambled – I did some of it with them – but knew nothing of the extent. Because I wasn't suffering obvious financial issues, because I was socially active, and because I honoured almost all my commitments, there was no reason for them to raise any concerns.

I was lying to them, though. I started to 'smoke bomb' – just completely disappear – from our nights out. I would say I'd gone home with a girl or had run into an old mate, but actually I was in the casino, normally for hours on end. Sometimes on the way to a social event I would go to the bookies or casino and then find myself stuck, trying to win back losses. I would arrive hours late or even not show at all.

I became increasingly unpredictable and occasionally there were consequences. One Friday, during a big day on the drink with work, I'd also lost a lot of money gambling. I headed home hammered and poor. I got in a cab and agreed a price with the driver to take me home – knowing full well that was all the cash I had.

When we pulled up outside my flat, the taxi driver charged me twice as much. I didn't have the money, lost my temper and refused to pay. As it turned out, one of my housemates (the one with whom I'd very much been burning the candle at both ends) had locked himself out of the flat. He was standing outside, waiting for someone to return, while eating a Domino's pizza. My housemate saw me hurling abuse at the driver and came to my rescue, taking my keys and letting me into the house while promising to return and settle up with the driver.

I stumbled upstairs and passed out, face down on my bed. But the cab driver had deemed my behaviour so appalling that he called the police. They arrived and, in my absence, arrested my housemate, who was taken to the police station and spent the night in a cell.

If it sounds like slapstick stuff, it wasn't, really. Having lost loads of money, I was angry and completely irrational. I was having violent reactions to gambling losses, and behaving in a manner that was totally unacceptable. Fortunately, my housemate could laugh about it before long and I was lucky that only he was there to see it.

Despite my lifestyle, I was still playing club cricket, and remained a very useful operator. After leaving uni I played for three teams around London. First, in the Surrey Championship with Spencer CC, with whom I reached the ECB National Knockout Final, then with Harpenden in 2009 and 2010. Halfway through 2010, I moved to play for Teddington in a very strong side that featured former England all-rounder Jamie Dalrymple, Aussie Big Bash player Josh Lalor and Dawid Malan, who went on to play Test cricket and become the No. 1 T20 batsman in the ICC rankings.

At Spencer, I'd been paid to play and coach. For the first time in my life, I wasn't playing cricket for the love of it; I was doing it for the money, because money funded my gambling.

At Teddington, I was known as a party animal but not as a gambler. I woke up one morning, when we were playing against Stanmore, to a load of missed calls. I had overslept and had to get straight in a cab to the game, which cost me about £100. The match had started at 11 a.m., but I'd only woken up at 11.05. By the time I arrived, the game was 18 overs in. The day before I'd been at Lord's for England's Test against Bangladesh, not that I'd watched much of it. I'd been drinking all day, into the pub afterwards, then onto the casino on my own, which was the secret reason I had overslept. This happened when I was at Harpenden, too. I was a good player, but I was a liability too.

My parents were aware that from time to time I struggled financially, but thought this came with the territory for a fun-loving youngster learning the ropes in an expensive city. They occasionally topped up my accounts to keep me afloat when, towards the end of the month, I said I needed a few extra quid because I was going on a holiday, a stag-do or needed some emergency dental treatment. They had no idea what they were funding.

When a rare moment of emotional vulnerability did surface, I was able to blame it on my break-up – I was still reeling from having my heart broken, I claimed. My ex and I had many mutual friends, which added another layer to the heartache because I didn't see some close mates for months. Nobody questioned this excuse when I was low.

But such glimpses of vulnerability were very rare. The deepening rut I was getting into was becoming apparent to me, but admitting mistakes wasn't going to happen. It was something that didn't come naturally to me because I'd little experience of it. I believed that accepting I had a rapidly developing problem would be a sign of weakness, and weakness wasn't something I did. I also feared others' reactions.

Financially, I was suddenly on a slippery slope. I first took out bank loans in February 2011. I was quite diligent with this initially, looking into interest rates, how much I was taking out, and the terms of the repayments. I did give it some consideration. But I was pretty desperate, and needed to open up a new revenue stream. I always intended to pay these off at the end of every month but it rarely happened. I'd pay a bit off, but never enough, not the full amount.

I also extended my overdraft from £1,000 to £2,500, and then again to £5,000 on 1 March – when I gambled away my whole month's salary (more than £2,000) in a single day. I had two credit cards, and there were two bank loans of £5,000 each.

That MCC tour to Hong Kong when I carried on like a millionaire? I took out a bank loan to afford that, just three months after winning enough money for a deposit on a house – a dream for someone who had just turned 24.

To cap six manic months that were pushing me towards breaking point, my appearance changed markedly too. The best part of 50 pints of lager and three doner kebabs or pizzas every week, becoming a proper smoker, dabbling in drugs, and barely sleeping meant that I looked very different to the professional athlete of just a few years before.

By June 2011, 18 hectic months into London life, I knew I had to act. I'd stopped enjoying my job and wanted a change. I decided insurance was boring but, most of all, I recognised that the culture at work wasn't helpful for a gambling addict and borderline alcoholic.

The question was, how much to divulge when revealing the reasons for a career change? My housemates – who didn't know I was being badgered by our landlord for failing to pay a month's rent – agreed a change would be a positive thing and accepted my decision to move on, so I headed to Sussex to speak to my parents. A consequence of my lifestyle was that I'd been – intentionally – speaking to them less and less. I'd always had a great relationship with them and used to speak to them often. But I'd been avoiding them because I knew that I was struggling and hated the idea of them, particularly my mum, worrying about me. They knew my life wasn't entirely plain sailing – they had seen my turmoil over the break-up, answered my requests for money and watched me pile on the pounds – but little more.

It was lovely to see them, as always. When I sat down for dinner, I decided to take the easy route. I went into detail about my need for change and disillusionment with London life, in particular how I didn't enjoy my job and struggled to keep up financially. I recalled my stint in teaching a couple of years earlier and said I wanted to follow them into that line of work long-term.

What I failed to mention was the gambling. I had about £12,500 debt, including being at the bottom of an extended £5,000 overdraft and taking out a series of bank loans, meaning I was struggling to pay my rent – which could have led to eviction. Leaving out these crucial but painful details meant, in my mind's eye, that I could move on with my life and the transition would be simpler. It also meant the conversation was easier, too.

They were extremely understanding about the mild struggles I'd shared, and ecstatic that my response was to get into teaching, which had brought them so much happiness and success over the years. The only questions they asked were how they could help me with the move.

Despite being on the verge of the summer holidays, my dad, widely respected in the teaching world, was confident that something could be in place by September. He started by helping me work on my CV – with my degree, time spent in the City and a stint as a professional cricketer I wasn't beyond hope – before making a few calls.

A few days later I was invited to an interview at a school in the heart of Oxford. It was a good school and had produced a number of famous faces in all sorts of fields down the years. It was also brilliantly located and had a youthful staff, so it ticked every box for me.

As I was shown around, my cricket career seemed as important as my credentials to teach history but, having answered questions about my willingness to get stuck into boarding life and my reasons for the move, I was offered a job from September. I wouldn't have an official title, but a position would be moulded for me. I was as keen as mustard, and felt I had a lot to offer. They weren't to know that I was immature and still getting to grips with adulthood and responsibility. Most 24-year-olds they employed were probably exactly the same.

I was taking a significant pay cut, although that was partially offset by being provided with accommodation. Less disposable income, I reasoned, might actually be a good thing right now. Convinced that this could be a watershed moment in my professional life, I accepted the position with glee and rushed back to London to finalise the move.

I requested a meeting with my boss first thing on Monday morning. Initially, he seemed furious I was leaving, assuming I was going to a competitor. But when I explained where I was going and 'why' (the truth and any tricky details were redacted once more), he was understanding. I would work another month, take a couple of weeks off, then hopefully use my new life to turn a corner.

5

August 2011

I loved my first year in teaching, and the move did me a lot of good.

I was entering an environment that, while new, I understood and felt comfortable in because I'd grown up in the schools my parents had worked in. The trouble I'd got myself into in London meant I arrived in Oxford apprehensive but hopeful that I could get my life back on track. It felt like a chapter of excess was closed. I was only 24, so I wasn't retreating to a monk-like existence. But I recognised that it had not taken me long to go off the rails in London, and plenty had to change.

In my new life, I wanted to gamble less. By leaving London, I'd recognised that I wasn't on the right track and that my gambling – with drink another factor – was an issue. It was unhealthy and even dangerous in the quantities I was doing it.

But that's not to say I wanted to quit. I knew I was doing it excessively but still felt that as something I enjoyed – at least when I won – it had a place in my life. The social element that had helped me fall in love with it was something I wanted to cling to, even if I was a long way past that. I wanted my relationship with gambling to return to the way it had been in the early days at Durham, where it had been so much fun and given me such a rush. It had just been part of my life, rather than a defining aspect. My belief was still that I was in control of all of this and could turn down the volume with ease. Why wouldn't I be able to do that? I was a strong guy with loads going for me. My ego was governing my behaviour again.

My new job was good for me. Choice was eliminated – or at least strongly minimised – from my life in a way that contrasted starkly with my London experience. Now, just as when I'd been a schoolboy, university student or academy cricketer, I was back in an institution with rules, timetables and the pressure of expectation from those around me. In this institution, as a teacher, I was in a position of responsibility. At once I was in my comfort zone – in a school – and out of my comfort zone – in a new role – and that combination meant I was duly institutionalised swiftly. I didn't want to put a foot wrong and was desperate to learn.

Living and working in a boarding school meant I didn't have as much exposure or access to the things that had caused problems in London, and essentially living with 60 adolescent boys – and being around many more kids all day long – was also a deterrent from all things naughty. Being around children for 12 or more hours every day, especially when you're not used to it, is not conducive to getting drunk and gambling. My week was quite literally timetabled down to every detail. I'd get half-an-hour's downtime here and there but even then, there was no hiding. I'd a one-bedroom flat in the boarding house, set between the gap-year students, who were doing all sorts of menial jobs that kept things ticking over, and the houseparents, who were in charge of the house. I was somewhere in between on the scale of authority and it all made for an interesting dynamic.

Part of the deal with the school was that I quite rightly had to get myself qualified as a teacher. In my second year I would be enrolled on a part-time PGCE training course at the University of Buckingham, but before the school were prepared to make that investment, I had to earn my stripes. I spent a huge amount of time observing lessons, planning how I would teach each one, and being observed myself by other members of staff.

I was essentially on trial. The school had taken a risk hiring me as I'd no teaching qualifications, so my contract was only for a year. I had to prove that I was worth a place on the course and at the school the following year. If not, it was back to the drawing board.

The things that pushed me to gamble were funds, time and boredom. Well, I lacked funds because the salary was low, and I lacked time because I was hectically busy. Being so busy and exploring new things also meant that I was never bored.

My new job was good for me in other regards beyond being a simple gambling deterrent. I quickly got to know my colleagues and made friends, meaning my social life was fun – and completely different to London. We would play five-a-side football or touch rugby, then nestle into a cosy pub. Only occasionally would we go out to a nightclub with the gap-year students, who were a bunch of fun-loving Aussies in their late teens, straight out of school. I'd stopped smoking because I was around children and I was drinking considerably less (although I could barely have been drinking much more in London). More exercise and less of the bad habits meant that I shifted some of the excess timber I'd put on in London and cut a healthier figure.

Generally, this was a far more active lifestyle. As a young teacher, there's not much standing still. In addition to my academic commitments I was outside coaching sports teams. In my spare time I played sport with my colleagues and in spring I joined a pair of clubs, first Frilford Heath, a local golf club, then Horspath Cricket Club. Most of my spare time in the next few months was spent at one of those two, particularly the golf club.

While work was bloody hard, I found the pace of life much less draining than it had been in London and I was sleeping much better – in part because I was getting into bed at a decent hour most days, and not staying up all hours drinking or staring at a screen gambling.

I was as busy as I'd ever been, and was feeling good about life and the decision I'd made the previous summer. I spent a lot of time working in the boarding house (a role which extended into the evening), coaching rugby and, while initially my time in the classroom was as a cover teacher, I was soon given responsibility to teach beginners' Latin after Christmas and welcomed the challenge.

That word I mentioned earlier – respect – was important too. I had to pay my dues at the school and in the profession that had served my family so well. I felt like I owed it to my parents to be on my best behaviour – the opposite of my London life. I was desperate to be a good teacher and to set myself on the path I'd follow for the rest of my career and life. In truth, I made a pretty good start.

Through juggling new friends and the responsibilities of pastoral care, coaching, planning, studying, marking and teaching, gambling took a backseat. Now, rather than having it on my doorstep, I had to drive to a bookies. It wasn't part of the culture of my workplace or friendship groups. None of my new mates gambled – or if they did, I didn't know about it – and I wasn't having conversations with them about gambling. As a result, I managed to limit my exposure to my vice. I deleted the gambling apps on my phone because I recognised that convenient accessibility was my biggest hazard; if I didn't have gambling at the end of my arm, I was bound to do it less. As a result, almost all my online gambling stopped. I wasn't using the fixed odds machines like I had been, and I definitely wasn't seeking out casinos.

I only bet at weekends, because that was when most sport was on. When I did, I wasn't betting anything like the stakes I used to because I didn't have the resources. My salary was too low, and I was trying to repair the financial damage I'd caused myself in London. I paid back some of the loans but never got close to paying any of them off in full. I could keep up with the repayments, but that left me with minimal disposable income and meant I couldn't save. Every penny was being used and I was in a tight spot.

That's not to say there weren't moments when I missed high-stakes gambling. And there was certainly temptation to go back to my old ways. But the lack of opportunities to gamble meant the windows of time required to manage that temptation were short. I resisted through some honest, old-fashioned willpower and the knowledge that I would still get my quiet little fix if I was able to on the weekend. I knew that stepping back was a good thing and I was on a better path than I'd been in London.

My financial situation improved slightly, as I paid back more of my debts, and so did my relationship with my family. We were working in the same field, so they were desperate to hear how I was getting on and I always had news to give them. I was more present and reliable, sticking to plans and not making excuses. It helped, too, that when I did speak to them, I was never asking for a few quid here and there to tide myself over after another loss. I could afford the life I was leading and the limited gambling I was engaging in.

If my relationship with my family improved, so did my relationships with my mates. Not only had I made new friends in Oxford, but I felt more relaxed about my social life with those I'd known for years. I had no ties to my ex in Oxford and, finally, I felt able to move on from that relationship, two years after it had ended. We had so many mutual friends that in London I felt constantly compromised, trying to avoid her and her friends at social engagements. The move to Oxford was a step away from that.

I missed my mates in London (and had a bit of FOMO once more) but got back there when I could. They recognised that I was in a considerably better place than I'd been the previous year. I was more measured in everything I did. I would still get hammered with them in town, but was a less manic, more reliable presence than I'd been. I wasn't suddenly disappearing or asking someone to loan me a hundred quid.

So, in the first few months until Christmas, I made real strides. But slowly things started to slide. On Boxing Day, a group of my uni mates had a tradition of going to Kempton Park Races for the King George VI Chase. I'd never been able to join them before but was free this year. Some of our closest family friends happened to be going, too. I was very much looking forward to a great day out.

Just because I'd dialled down my gambling didn't mean the passion for racing I'd developed in recent years had dwindled. I still kept tabs on form, followed tipsters online, checked results, read the *Racing Post* when I could and had a very occasional punt on horses that I particularly liked. As well as being picky about my horses, I would also stick to the big races and meets rather than betting on any and every race going, as I had when in the bookies around Lloyd's. I'd only placed a handful of bets on racing in my time in Oxford.

The racing card on Boxing Day provided more than enough to satisfy me after what felt a long time away. My favourite horse, Kauto Star, was running in the main event, bidding for a fifth win in the King George. He was up against Long Run, a young pretender and the favourite, meaning Kauto Star was available at odds of 3/1 – unheard of! Another of my favourite horses, Binocular, was being ridden by AP McCoy in the Grade One Christmas Hurdle. I was looking forward to seeing my friends, but I was also looking forward to the sport we were attending.

I was, by my standards of the time, quite flush with cash on Boxing Day 2011. I'd been home with my parents for a couple of weeks since term had ended, limiting my spending, and I'd received some cash for Christmas.

Given Kauto Star's generous odds I decided to back him, and to place a double with Kauto Star and Binocular, as well as in a treble with Grand Crus, ridden by Tom Scudamore, in the other Grade One race that day. I considered this a Christmas treat to myself after months of good behaviour.

All three came through and I won over £11,000, from a relatively small stake – it wasn't like in London when I'd put £500 on. Everyone else had backed Kauto Star too, so we had a great time celebrating. Using an old trick, I kept the scale of my winnings private and, when asked, said that I'd won about a grand. No one batted an eyelid; I think a few of my mates had done pretty well, too.

Needless to say, this changed things for me in the following days, weeks and months – but not as radically as the £35k win had the previous December. I started to gamble more often than I had been, and my stakes rose. It gave me another taste for winning and that sense of invincibility I'd had before, the belief that another big win was round the corner.

But I'd worked hard enough to turn myself around in the previous few months that I didn't see this purely as free money to be gambled away. I wouldn't have been able to pay the punchy joining fee at the golf club, which was due after Christmas, without using money from my win. I paid off some of my credit card debt, and cleared my overdraft. I'd been on the right track in terms of fixing the significant financial damage I'd done in London, and this went further towards helping the situation. This was clearly a positive step but ominously it now meant that I felt I had some financial slack.

Back at school, my focus remained strongly on teaching and my new life. I wasn't suddenly reckless. I still lacked time to gamble excessively and had been relatively sensible with my money. But little habits did start to creep back in. I began to fill little pockets of time – when my timetable allowed – with gambling on my phone, where I'd re-installed the bookies' apps.

One example was when I was on 'dorms duty', which was essentially looking after the boys in the evening, sending them to bed and turning the lights off at 9 p.m. From then, the on-duty teacher was required to hang around for an hour or so to check they were quiet, rather than chatting all night, having pillow-fights and all the other hi-jinks teenage boys get up to. In my first term, I diligently planned lessons and sports sessions in this time, or tied up other loose ends. But after Christmas, I would sit down in the corridor outside the dorm, get out my phone and bet on football or play casino games. It wasn't excessive, but it was corrosive.

As in my first term, I didn't feel the need to go to the bookies. But that didn't mean I couldn't gamble. Some of the Boxing Day winnings were plonked into my online account, so I just needed my phone to hand. Now, though, on the occasions when I did go into town, I might pop into the bookies as discreetly as I possibly could. I lived in absolute fear that I would be seen going into the shop by a parent, a colleague, a teacher at another school (I was getting to know them through sports matches) or, perhaps worst of all, a pupil. So, my visits were rare and generally brief. I got back into having a couple of spins on the fixed odds machines again, but was sensible enough to recognise it had to be exactly that – a couple of spins – rather than a whole afternoon sat in the bucket chair.

I did also start to make a few 'bigger' bets again, on what I considered 'dead certs'. I gave myself a weekly budget of £250 for gambling. Most of the time I stuck to it, though sometimes I didn't. The lofty ambition was to turn that £250 into £1,000, which was obviously difficult; it was also difficult to have the discipline to withdraw money from my online account when I won. The stakes weren't on the scale of my London days and the odds were very short; essentially, I saw this attitude to betting as a tactical move to pay off my debts. Most of the bets came through, as the odds suggested they should. But, of course, not all of them did, and the trouble was that when I did lose I immediately tried to win the money back.

So my second and third terms as a teacher weren't as squeaky clean as my first. But I wasn't in the self-destructive mode I'd been in while living in London, and my general behaviour was infinitely better. My socialising was healthier, my commitment to, and performance in, my job were both high, and I was happy.

In my much-improved family life, it helped that my sister, who's three years older than me, got married in April 2012. My new brother-in-law had been on the scene for years, and I got on brilliantly with him. The build-up to that event helped give my life a family focus, and it was an amazing day on the Sussex Downs. In that moment, my London troubles felt a lifetime away and I felt an immensely happy, lucky bloke.

I was asked to MC the wedding and enjoyed the day hugely. It took place on 14 April, the same day as the Grand National at Aintree. It's little surprise that in this role I took it upon myself to organise a sweepstake with the male half of the wedding party – my dad, brother, my brother-in-law's family and his ushers. The race was an absolute classic, with Neptune Collonges beating Sunnyhill Boy in a photo finish, the tightest finish ever in the 165-year history of the event. Typically, I'd drawn Sunnyhill Boy in the sweepstake. As MC, I announced the result to the room through gritted teeth because, as ever, I could have done with the money and hated losing. It would have taken a far bigger stake than a few quid to ruin a wonderful day, though.

Around that time, I started playing cricket for Horspath as a new season had begun. The school gave me Saturdays off to play and I quickly embraced the club's ethos and attitude. We were a little club in a village outside Oxford with a great tight-knit feel and aspirations to rise up the leagues and face the big boys.

I was, in effect, their first 'marquee signing' who had played at a higher level and I immediately slotted in. I was very well looked after; I wasn't paid to play – no one was, except for the overseas pro – but the club didn't make me pay subs and funded my kit, too. The standard was good, the club was upwardly mobile with a lot of talented young guys, and I enjoyed playing again. The team ethic at the club was as strong as any I've ever been a part of.

Away from the ripples caused by the Boxing Day blip was another lapse – a few short-lived flings on the teaching scene locally. Boarding schools are small, intense places, and very little goes unnoticed. Everything was secret, and quite audacious, which appealed to my risk-taking instincts. None of these relationships lasted long, but I probably did take too many risks.

And as I gambled a bit more, my general behaviour became looser and bolder. I went out more. I led a less healthy existence too. By other teachers, and especially my superiors, I was seen as reliable and enthusiastic, a very professional new teacher who always said 'yes' and threw himself into every task. Yet the gap-year students and other younger staff saw me increasingly as a party animal and a joker. I knew there were aspects of my behaviour that were a little unprofessional but I wanted to have it both ways.

And then my first summer holidays arrived.

6

July 2012

Normally, the end of the summer term is nirvana for teachers. Indeed the ample, hard-earned holidays – with the summer the jewel in the crown – are a reason some do the job. Friends in other professions looked on green-eyed as I embarked on the two-month break at the end of my first year, from early July through to early September.

The end of my first year arrived rather suddenly. Obviously, I knew when the holidays were starting and could see the end of term coming but by the end of any school year even the most experienced teacher is run off their feet and utterly knackered. It's a time of reports, deadlines and logistics that occupy you right up to the moment the last kids walk out of the gate. When they did, I suddenly thought, 'Right, what now?'

Having been operating at a million miles an hour all year, suddenly I had nothing to do. Time stood still, and I felt a sense of loss. I wasn't completely bereft of things to do. I still played plenty of sport. I had a cricket match every Saturday with Horspath and we trained on Tuesday and Thursday evening. Occasionally we had a midweek match, too. I played golf at Frilford whenever I could with whoever would play with me. I went away on holiday with my family.

But that only filled so many hours in the week and so many weeks in the summer. I was single and lived alone in a small flat in a now-deserted school. Many of my new friends spent the summer out of Oxford with their partners or kids, catching up after an arduous academic year in the school bubble. I missed not having a partner with whom I could naturally fill my spare time, and give and receive affection. I was envious of mates who were in that position. Put simply, I was lonely. And time alone didn't come naturally to me.

Not being at work also cost me a lot more money. Whereas in term time I could eat school meals with colleagues or the kids, I now had to pay for my food. And in term time, when working hard, indulging hobbies was rarely possible, saving me more money and meaning the pay cut I'd taken wasn't as much of an issue. That summer, I needed both more stimulation and more cash.

So, I spent much of my time in one of three places: Betfred on the Marston Ferry Road, Ladbrokes in Summertown, or on the sofa in my flat. In the first two, my activities were obvious. From the sofa, I would flick through any sport my TV or laptop could offer me with my phone in hand, relentlessly logging in to Paddy Power's online offering.

I struggled to conquer the challenges that loneliness and the subsequent boredom posed. I fell back into gambling, using it as a comfort blanket and a companion. Whole days would pass, sat in a bucket chair at Betfred, which I only left to pop to the Co-op for a quick sandwich. I was back betting on my old staples – racing, roulette, cricket and golf – but even that didn't keep me busy enough. I spent even more time reading the *Racing Post*, studying form and trying to strategically plan my bets. And, when the betting shops shut at 9 p.m., I explored the world of online gambling ever more aggressively.

I could now gamble at any time, in any place, on any device. I'd gambled online before but it had always been a bit on the side, just part of the package. Now it became central. My gambling online came in three forms across a number of different accounts – maybe half a dozen – that I flitted between. There was the gambling that I'd done before (which was essentially the same as what I would do in a betting shop – casino games and betting on sport), then there was the Betfair Exchange, and spread betting through the likes of Sporting Index.

I had never used the Exchange or done spread betting before. I came across them through adverts on TV while watching sport and more targeted advertising on social media, and was especially attracted by introductory deals that tempted me to open new accounts. Social media became an ever-greater part of my gambling, and also alerted me to new ways to bet as I followed what others were talking about. I followed eagerly every tip and suggestion.

I loved spread betting because it allowed me to gamble 'in play', and you could (in essence) buy and sell. You would bet on whether a specific outcome during the game was above or below a spread – the range within which the result will fall – offered by the betting company. How much you won or lost would depend on how far above or below the spread the outcome finished at.

The spread has a 'buy' price at the top, and a 'sell' price at the bottom. You would buy if you thought the outcome would be more than the spread, and sell if it would be below. For instance, in a football match, the spread could be set at 2.8 to 3.2, if those setting it believed there were likely to be three goals in the match. If I thought there'd be four, I'd 'buy' big. If I thought there'd only be one, I'd 'sell'. And if things weren't going your way once the game got underway, you could bet against what you originally had.

I would bet on cricket particularly, gambling on every single dismissal and player's involvement. There was an outcome to every single delivery. It was great for racing too. I could back a horse before a race, then back it again while it was running. Equally, I could 'lay', which was essentially selling back the bet to the bookie. I loved the sense that it was constantly evolving and that it involved me – the competition was constant.

Needless to say, you could win big money quickly, and lose it rapidly too. There was even more risk and reward, which satisfied my need for instant gratification. The race or game never seemed to be over – there was always new hope to be found. And there were simply so many markets that everything in the game began to matter. I could bet on smaller elements like the number of corners in a football match, and would suddenly be invested in the ball going out of play.

Within all this, I had my personal quirks. I would back games to be high scoring – runs in cricket, goals in football, points in rugby – in the hope that it would produce an entertaining and profitable game. I would back against teams I supported or players I particularly liked so it was win-win if they did well. The blow of losing money – which I was doing plenty of – was softened by the success of my team.

A few months later, in November, I stayed up most of the night to watch and bet on the first Test of Australia's home summer series against South Africa at the Gabba in Brisbane. At this stage, I wasn't an insomniac, but I definitely didn't sleep much.

In their first innings, South Africa racked up a massive score, so it was clearly a great pitch for batting. I decided to back Ricky Ponting, the legendary Australia batsman, hard. He'd come into the game showing great form and had been a class player for 15 years. I bought him at £10 per run. His spread would have been something between 40 and 50 runs, so every run he scored over that, I would win big. If he didn't make it to 40, I was in trouble.

Ponting was dismissed for a duck – a disastrous outcome that lost me £400 straight off the bat (well, the edge of the bat as he was caught at second slip). And to make matters worse, I started to chase my losses. Because Ponting was out and Australia were in trouble, I decided to bet heavily against Michael Clarke – who had replaced Ponting as captain the year before and at the crease in that innings – on the basis that South Africa would remain on top. Well, they didn't. Clarke came out and made 259 not out, the third of four double-centuries he made in 2012, the best year of a very good career. Meanwhile, Ponting retired two matches later as his 38th birthday approached. Betting on that game, everything that could have gone wrong for me did – but it didn't stop me doing more, despite having lost more than £1,000 by the close of play. Needless to say, this was an extremely addictive form of gambling.

I also got into the Betfair Exchange, which is effectively a gambling market place. You would either back an outcome or 'lay' it – essentially betting on it not happening. There are odds, but they're presented as a decimal rather than a fraction (odds of 2/1 would be 3.0 and 3/1 would be 4.0, and so on). The direction the rest of the market was heading would set the odds, not the bookmaker themselves.

Again, this form of gambling could be brilliant or disastrous. The risk of laying was huge – and I would lay all the time. I would lay the favourite in a horse race so if any other horse won the race, I would win.

This also involved plenty of betting in-play, which was awful for anyone with a developing gambling problem. It used to be that you would place your bet at the start of an event and that was that, you would sit back and wait for the result. But now I would sit there analysing whether to cash out if things were going well or badly as the event unfolded. If I delayed a decision to cash out by just a few seconds, I could win extra money without anything changing because the odds constantly changed in-play. But if things did change for the worse in that short period – for instance, if a team I'd not backed scored a goal – I would suffer very heavy losses.

Things developed in other ways. Over the course of my first year at the school I'd established that one of my closest colleagues was also sports mad, liked the occasional punt and followed the horses. Gambling wasn't a big part of his life, so despite quickly becoming friends, it took a while to come up in conversation.

It turned out he followed a couple of tipsters online (I followed every tipster under the sun) and would occasionally act on one of these tips, putting a fiver on here and there, nothing more. He was the only person I ever discussed gambling with at school, and before too long, he introduced me to a mate of his who was a professional gambler.

There are lots of professional gamblers about, although not many would necessarily use that term to describe their occupation. There are professional poker players as well as those who 'trade' on sports – mainly using the Betfair Exchange. To them, sport is a series of events to be traded like stocks and shares.

I was invited to take part in a mutually beneficial scheme the pro had with a few of his friends, and friends of friends. Because he won a lot, he would regularly have his accounts shut down by online bookmakers, who thought they detected suspicious betting patterns or insider trading. This meant he had to get inventive to keep gambling, and keep making money.

So, he would ask a mate to set up an account, into which he would deposit, say £1,000. They would put in 10 per cent of whatever he did, and hand over the login details. When he was finished with the account – normally because it got closed down – he would hand his mate 10 per cent of his winnings, which was often a significant sum.

He was constantly on the lookout for new people to help him out in what should have been a low-maintenance way of earning extra cash. I would come to know this guy a little bit over the next few years, but when I first got involved, we had only met a couple of times. We exchanged a few WhatsApps here and there, but we didn't have much to do with each other.

There was a big difference between the relationship with my mate from school and the one I had with the professional. My mate put his money in and let the pro do his stuff. As a result, he made money and was successful. In fact, he still does to this very day. When term began again, he would talk to me about it at school, saying how well we were doing and what a great system it was. I would nod along in agreement – but things weren't going quite as well for me.

My mate had no idea of the scale of my gambling. Based on the conversations we had, he would have thought that, like him, I enjoyed a punt because I loved sport. It was an opportunity for me, like him, to make a few extra quid. Every now and again, for fun, he might log into the online account to see how the pro was getting on, just to bring a smile to his face when he learned that a grand had grown twelvefold. He was in line for £1,200 of it.

By contrast, I was logging on regularly and would certainly not just settle for taking my cut. I would watch closely what the professional was doing, and then try to replicate it independently. So, I'd see that he'd put £1,000 on Kolkata Knight Riders to hit more sixes than Mumbai Indians in the IPL, and when it happened, I'd double my money. Very nice.

But I was too greedy, and enjoyed it too much. I'd place the same bet in the second innings of a game or the next time that team played, even if the pro hadn't bet on it, and I'd lose. Or I'd see his next bet and put on 10 times the amount he had, and it would be one of his rare losses. His loss would be manageable for him, part of what he was in the business of doing (he couldn't win every time, or we'd all be doing it). My loss, on the other hand, was disastrous.

Watching the huge money he made, I started to wonder whether I could go down the same route. I would suggest that most gambling addicts have this moment (normally after a big win, when everything seems so easy) when they believe they could do it professionally. I genuinely thought about it. Why not make the thing I loved most my job? This guy is doing it. I have no idea what the pro earned, but it would have been plenty more than me.

What stopped me taking it any further wasn't the fact that I would have been truly terrible at it, but my view of gambling. I was ashamed of my habit, and couldn't abide the idea of telling people (starting with my parents) that I gambled for a living. I thought gambling was fundamentally wrong, which is strange given I did it so much.

I would have been a hopeless pro. In the way we gambled, the pro and I could barely have been more different. He was as dispassionate as I was impulsive. He used his head, I followed my heart. For him, it was functional, for me it was a fix.

He bet mainly on cricket, because that was what he knew the most about and followed most closely, but he didn't gamble relentlessly. He would target very specific bets that he thought were good value and very likely to happen. If he bet on how many runs were scored in the first six overs of a game, that could be his only bet of the whole match. He would settle for that because he might not have been confident enough to place any other bet, which was all informed by research, form, statistics and knowledge – right down to how the weather radar was looking. Clearly, I did not bet in this way.

Occasionally, we crossed paths and I'd get a look at him in action. A mutual friend got married and we went on the stag do together, which involved a trip to Epsom races. In contrast to cricket, he really knew very little about racing, so didn't take any risks. I remember finding it absolutely extraordinary that this professional gambler was putting just a few quid on at the races, while I was hiding my betting slips with much higher stakes. He was so measured and calculated.

As an aside, that stag do was also an example of the state of my gambling at this time. The stag party came together to put a huge group bet on a horse. We pooled all the kitty money, and a lot of lads backed the same horse independently too. It was one of those moments where, if we won, the stag do goes to a whole other level.

I obviously put my share into the kitty. But I'd had a tip from a guy I knew who was involved in horse racing to back a different horse in the same race. I just couldn't resist putting big money on that horse, too.

Inevitably, the group horse won and mine didn't even place. All the lads were buzzing with the big win, going mental. I tried to do the same but had lost a huge amount of money – in excess of £1,000. I kept that to myself and made it through the day, with a lot of alcohol. The next day I was in pieces.

My approach to gambling just didn't fit with the pro's. It meant I couldn't keep up with him; there were times when he asked me to set up another account with the same 10 per cent deal, but I simply didn't have the money to get involved. When I did make money with him, I just reinvested it to fund my addiction. Just like the mate who introduced us, I have no doubt that if the pro knew how much I was gambling he wouldn't have let me get involved in the first place.

Gambling online made things feel more secretive, and a little more illicit. In a shop, there was some camaraderie and atmosphere, lots going on. While I never had anyone I would call a friend in the bookies, there were still regulars I would talk gambling with and celebrate wins with. I'd know the staff behind the counter, and there were some shops I preferred going to because of who worked in them.

I also liked the feeling of actually having cash in your hands because that made it feel real – it was my money – and therefore I would tend to lose less. Online it just felt like numbers on a screen, and any semblance of control was lost.

I might have been entertained, but the summer of 2012 was a devastating one financially. Sat alone on my sofa, any notion of gambling being a shared activity was gone. It was this summer too that, when I did things away from my sofa, I started gambling alongside them on my phone. When I played golf, I was constantly on my phone (which is rude, a bad look, and frankly impractical), gambling or checking scores. When I played cricket and was waiting to bat, I'd be doing the same. When we were fielding, the first thing I'd do when I got in for the lunch or tea break was to check my phone to see how things were going. Sometimes I couldn't even wait that long and would field on the boundary, asking those watching what the football scores were. My mind was on my phone, not the game. And when I went away with my family, I was glued to my phone and spent plenty of time in the only really private place in our holiday home – the toilet.

The cycle returned. There were times when I won big, but when I lost, I would chase big wins and make the situation worse. I would be back on the phone to the bank, asking for an overdraft extension, usually lying about funding an imaginary holiday or having to replace a car. I still had a reasonable credit rating because I paid off credit cards sporadically so appeared a viable customer for banks, who were willing to lend to me. I was able to top up previous loans on repayment terms that appeared manageable, and I got my hands on a couple of credit cards with sizeable limits. I lived exclusively at the bottom of my overdraft, except for a day or two after I received my salary. The idea of having a lower salary being a good thing as it put a brake on my gambling was now a distant memory. My salary no longer limited my gambling.

After such a promising year, I'd taken a massive turn for the worse – in no time at all. I'd spent the six months since Boxing Day gambling more, but (by my standards) still in moderation. I felt in control, I gambled when I wanted to, and other things in my life came first. I'd shown that I was able to adapt to my new working life and change my behaviour very quickly. I dialled down my gambling when I started teaching. Habits, good and bad, came easily to me. And with time on my hands over the summer holidays, I allowed myself to drift into bad habits faster than ever.

But when the summer holidays ended, this serious turn for the worse couldn't simply be solved by a return to school. I'd been looking forward to the start of term, to the routine, the distraction, the company and the camaraderie that I'd missed all summer.

Throughout my first year in teaching, I'd not had the time or opportunity to gamble as heavily as I had been. I'd been focused on a tough new challenge. But the compulsion to gamble more still lay within me, waiting, not far from the surface. I'd done nothing to address that. When I'd left London, I'd lied about the true reasons and hoped that a big change would see my issues drift away. I hoped that I could pack my bags, change my habits and that would be that. It worked, for a bit. But the roots ran deeper than that and, having not taken any concrete steps to rid myself of my need to gamble, it was only ever a matter of time before it rose to the surface once more. It's easy enough to see now that I needed professional help, but I was still far from seeking it – or acknowledging how big my problem was.

That's partly because I knew nothing about gambling addiction and definitely didn't consider myself an addict. I knew alcoholics – in fact, I was close to being one – and I knew people who liked drugs a bit too much. But I wasn't aware of any gambling addicts. Even footballers from the 1990s, like Paul Merson, who we now know was a gambling addict, were presented as rogues who liked a fag, a beer, a line and a punt. In the little I'd seen or read, there was something almost glamorous about it, a far cry from the increasingly sinister experience I was going through.

Over the summer, I became so gripped by gambling that I couldn't prevent it forcing its way into my working life when school resumed in September. My level of debt had increased over the holidays, so my constant gambling was also an attempt to pay that off. Moving online meant I could gamble anywhere and while I was doing other things. I'd spent my first year becoming accustomed to life and school. I'd started to understand the job and its rhythms. Now, I just fitted gambling into every lull. I wasn't safe from my addiction during the school day.

As the new term began, I found myself sat at my computer planning lessons or marking books, as I bet on – and watched – horse racing. I was a master of the multitask. It was convenient for me, too, that it was around this time that teachers were expected to be 'on call' a little bit more – answering emails from parents, pupils and colleagues on our phones while on the move.

In my job, I now had increased responsibility and a PGCE to complete, but my concern wasn't teaching a full timetable, my studies or various other new roles, it was balancing that with my constant compulsion to gamble. I was, by now, very good at hiding what I was doing. When I needed to put on a work face, I could. When I needed to put on a brave face after a tough loss, I could. When I needed to put my phone down for a bit, I could. No one noticed. The trouble was that beneath the surface, I was beginning to drown.

You may have noticed that I'm now referring to myself as a gambling addict. There's no moment in my mind that sticks out as a specific marker of my deep problem, but a little over a year after my move to teaching I could no longer control my need to bet. But I was in denial about that need.

Once more, there was no chance of me admitting that I was being overwhelmed financially and physically. I feared admitting mistakes, having tough conversations and letting people down. I was convinced that I could break free myself, with that one big win.

Despite all my problems, for the next couple of years, I cruised. Very luckily, nothing disastrous happened as a result of my gambling addiction. You hear the term 'functioning alcoholic' a lot. Well, I was a functioning gambling addict.

We talk about drug addicts needing 'a hit'. I needed a hit, too. But at this time, a hit would tide me over for a decent amount of time. I was gambling a lot, but I was gambling around my life. I was able to put bets on in the morning before work, then get through the day teaching, ticking boxes and appearing respectable. If I was busy, I wouldn't feel the need to check how things were going or to place more bets. I would bet again when I was next able to, whether that was in a free period, the lunch break, or when I finally got into bed in my one-bed flat that night.

But there were moments when I let my guard drop and made mistakes. On one occasion I was supposed to be going on the school ski trip. Staff going on the trip had to pay a contribution. One Saturday I was in London and convinced myself that I could go to the casino and fund my trip in one sitting. I got myself about £5,000 up (more than five times what I actually needed), then got greedy and lost it all – and more (approximately what the trip would have cost me). That night, I got on the bus back to Oxford absolutely devastated. I arrived home and went straight to the pub and drowned my sorrows.

At one Cheltenham Festival, by now established as an annual highlight for me, things went very wrong. I was supposed to be at work on the Friday, which was the day of the Gold Cup, but managed to persuade the school to give me the day off by claiming I needed to attend a stag do. School obliged and some mates came to stay in my flat on Thursday evening before we headed west early on the Friday.

As ever, we drank hard, spending most of the day in the Guinness Village. I'd put a huge bet on a horse owned by a parent of a kid I'd taught. Just before the race, one of my best mates and

I were making our way back to the grandstand from our station in the Guinness Village. On the way, we were interrupted by a woman giving out scarves as part of her promotional work for Betfair. We took one and, after a very crass attempt to chat her up, I asked who her tip for the same race was. She said Lord Windermere, which I laughed off. Deep down, though, I became absolutely intent on putting money on that horse. I couldn't bear the thought of receiving a recommendation and not acting on it.

My phone, at this point, was plugged in at a charging station elsewhere, so I couldn't use it to bet, and the crowds were too heavy for us to make it to the tote in time to back the horse. I never did put that bet on and, of course, Lord Windermere breezed home as an outsider. I was distraught and turned to the booze, as usual.

A couple of hours later I could be seen outside the Veuve Clicquot tent doing a striptease – which had become a very embarrassing party trick that I could be cajoled into doing by my mates (I always wanted to be seen as the most fun person at the party) – for a very smart middle-aged woman I'd never met before. The police approached and I began to push my luck, providing a policewoman with the same tease (which saw me horsing around in my boxer shorts, despite it being March), with a big crowd watching on in hysterics. The police, patience running thin, gave me a warning, so I got dressed and was thrown out of the tent to a rapturous round of applause. I was absolutely battered, way beyond control, and had spent a huge amount of money. All I could think about was Lord Windermere. Over the next two days, I spent almost every minute trying to win back the money I thought was rightly mine, and suffered devastating losses.

Generally, though, things weren't as dramatic as that. I functioned by leading a very tiring life in which I never stopped moving. I'd always been an efficient worker, but I now took it to a new level. I would get up earlier than I needed to, about 6 a.m., and be working immediately to get a teacher's menial tasks – planning, marking and other admin – out of the way as fast as I could. I would respond to emails promptly, manage things at breakneck speed and, actually, be very good at the job in hand. Those around me thought I was organised, efficient and committed. I was even promoted, which meant I had a host of new responsibilities on the pastoral and sports side. I was also doing my PGCE, so had essays to write and lots of lessons to observe.

By lunchtime, I'd usually cleared my work and could pop to the bookies and get my hit. In the afternoon, I could watch and bet on horse racing on my phone around my other commitments. If work was done a bit early, say by 5 p.m., I could pop to the bookies or continue gambling at home. And in the evening, I could watch football without thinking about my job.

Paradoxically, the deeper the gambling hole I dug for myself, the more efficient I became at school – in the knowledge that I was doing something wrong in my private life, I had to make my guard completely impenetrable. I didn't want to be questioned. A perfect example was that at the end of the year I received an Outstanding grade on my PGCE, despite everything that was going on. I was quite brilliant at hiding what I needed to hide.

Inevitably, I occasionally also had moments when I let myself down. After a night on the beers or a trip to London and the casino, I would sometimes oversleep, missing assemblies or occasionally even a lesson. I tried to make excuses, but they were never very good – simply that I'd overslept, or something similarly unsophisticated. I did try and plan ahead though. I would arrange cover or make excuses in advance to allow myself some leeway. This was particularly relevant for my lessons on a Saturday morning (many boarding schools have lessons then);

I was lucky that I had a good mate who was usually happy to swap with me. I never found myself in trouble with the school, but these little slips didn't go totally unnoticed either.

With all this going on, there were elements of my life that I just couldn't keep up with. In 2013, I stopped enjoying playing cricket, my lifelong passion. I liked being involved at Horspath because of the social life and the great group of lads I played with. I was playing other games too, including my MCC qualifying matches (play a certain number and you become a member at Lord's) but I saw them as a chore rather than a pleasure or an honour, which they should have been. I should have been playing Minor Counties cricket (the level below full-time professional) regularly for Oxfordshire and did play one game that summer. But my attitude wasn't right. I had little interest, because my mind was elsewhere. Having wanted to be a cricketer for so long, I was now spurning the opportunity to play at a high level. For some reason I seemed to think it was beneath me, which it definitely wasn't.

Socially, my relationships with friends suffered and I lost touch with many. If I wasn't directly involved with someone, if they weren't an immediate priority, I drifted from them.

I felt guilty, too, that I was beginning to become more socially unreliable, which meant strained relationships with good friends who were important to me. I would still get invited to London but my attendance was increasingly hit and miss. Friends of mine who were still there were also increasingly becoming high rollers, and the thought of going to join them, and dropping £200 on a big day and night of fun was increasingly impossible.

There were times when I was on my way to the train or bus station to get to London, and would pop into the bookies to try to win the cost of my night out. I'd inevitably lose money, hit the bottom of the overdraft, and have to turn round and go back home. I made my excuses and would say I couldn't come because something had suddenly come up at work, but people started to notice.

None of my friends realised how much I gambled. A few of them, as they always had, liked a bet, and we were all in WhatsApp groups where we'd talk about gambling. But they had no sense of how much I was doing it. If we were betting on something I lumped on so much more cash than any of them, and so much more often, too.

I didn't have a relationship of any permanence. To me, this meant I didn't have to keep up appearances in my flat, which was very much my own space and, frankly, a total mess. In many ways it was my gambling den.

I'd become an extremely secretive person. As a result, I felt increasingly isolated, and could feel the walls closing in on an ever-more troubled life. At boarding school, it's hard to do anything at all without everyone in the community knowing about it. There are positives to a tight-knit community, but it's claustrophobic and can be suffocating.

The fact that I was living a double life, never confiding in anyone else, made it a nightmare. I'd to be on my guard at all times. It was made more complicated by the fact that my sister (working in the learning support department) and her husband joined the school in my second year and, a year after that, my brother joined another local school as a junior teacher, too. I was very close to all three, and on the surface this was great news for my life in Oxford.

But my sister and her husband would be right on my doorstep, so I was torn. They're a bit older than me and I'd always had a great relationship with both of them. I'd never argued or fought with my sister, and at times we had been so close that she'd seemed like a second mother. She'd supported me through homesickness at boarding school, she'd acted as an unofficial relationship counsellor, and had always been a voice of reason and pillar of solidity in my life. She's brilliantly caring and kind, and has always put others' interests in front of her own. My brother-in-law is someone I got on with from the moment my sister had first introduced him to the family a few years earlier. We clicked immediately and he was someone I considered a good friend.

It was a big move for them to come to Oxford, and I didn't want to stand in their way or deny them a great opportunity, but I had my reservations about them joining. My brother-in-law, just as I had a year earlier, was making a considerable career change, and it was obviously a big step in their life, having only got married a few months earlier. He was actually slotting into exactly the same role at the school that I had held the previous year.

But Oxford, and indeed the school, had become my patch, I'd made friends and a life for myself there. Of course, my sister and her husband were brilliant when they joined and, not wanting to tread on my toes, they just got stuck into their new jobs.

But with them so close by, I had to be even more careful not to give away that I was getting myself into serious financial and emotional trouble. I would see them every day so had to present a strong front, giving the impression that everything was well, so that this would be the message relayed to my parents – who I'd reverted to talking to less and less.

When my brother joined us all in Oxford a year later, it was a bit different. He was straight out of uni and went to work at a school nearby. We met up about twice a week. As he was at a different school I didn't have to worry about whispers about my behaviour at school like I did with my sister.

It helped that my brother and I, who were best mates in many ways, would meet up to do things I liked. We would play sport – squash, golf, or 5-a-side football with other teachers – and get on the beers. Time with him was a distraction from my troubles.

If nothing was going terribly wrong publicly, my finances began to slip further out of control. When I first gambled at uni,

I'd used my student loan, my allowance and my cricket salary. In London, I'd had a proper income for the first time. When I lost control there, after blowing my big win, I'd taken out bank loans and signed up for credit cards. But there are only so many times you can do that before the banks and creditors start saying 'no'.

My finances fluctuated wildly from month to month. Good months would tide me over for some time. To keep gambling, I had to win a lot, and I did. I wasn't completely hopeless at it, and my love and interest in sport meant I had a keen eye for a good bet.

One of the issues was that when I won big on sport, I'd turn to casino games, which were much more about luck than judgement, to get my fix. Pair that with the vicious nature of spread betting, where I'd win and lose big, and trouble was never far away.

So there were bad months. And for the first few of those, I asked my mum and dad for a bit of cash to tide me over and they agreed. I blamed it on a financial hangover from my time in London. Eventually, though, I couldn't ask them any more. For starters, they were generous, but didn't have an endless supply. More importantly, I didn't want to raise their suspicions.

I asked a couple of mates for money, too. They were generally older and able to afford to lend me £500 or so, which I would pay back over the following months. But by the end of 2013, my loans were as big as they could be, so banks would no longer lend to me, and my credit cards were maxed out. As I became more desperate, I turned to payday loans. I could do this, I reasoned, because I was only ever a win away from sorting them out. I was one accumulator away from a magic wand being waved.

The first was with a company called Pounds to Pocket, for £1,500, which I was supposed to pay back by the end of the month. Unsurprisingly, I ended up making only a minimum payment, accruing interest at eye-watering rates, which quickly became a theme.

Soon enough I'd taken out loans with Wonga, QuickQuid, Bongaloans, PayDayAdvance, Peachy, Sunny, Wageday Advance – anyone who would lend to me. Repaying them was never as simple as I'd hoped it would be; there were times I would have the cash at the start of the month, but others when I'd gambled too much and had nothing left.

During 2014, I borrowed more off friends than I ever had before. It was little and often, and I was much better at paying them back than the payday loans companies or banks. While this meant relationships remained intact, it was very bad news in terms of the interest that built up on my other borrowing. Some of these payday loans had an Annual Percentage Rate (APR) of 500 per cent.

My desperation for cash was evident in other ways. If I was given a cheque as a gift or for a service (such as cricket coaching), I couldn't afford to wait the five days it took for it to land in my account, so I would cash it there and then, even though I got charged 10 per cent of the amount for the privilege. If had anything of worth to sell, I'm sure I would have done, but I didn't; I was heading into my late 20s with no assets or savings, just a load of debt. Friends were buying houses and making investments, but I couldn't begin to think about that.

Also in 2014, I began running coaching courses in the school holidays. They were very successful and the uptake was excellent, with parents looking to keep their kids busy during the holidays (they didn't realise that I really needed keeping busy, too). My brother would help out on some of them, unaware that I wasn't seeing a penny of the good wedge of cash we were taking home – I was using it all to keep my head above water.

All of my spending was linked to my addiction. My income went on betting (and drinking), or paying off debts and meeting repayment commitments; and by not meeting those I was only deepening the trouble. Occasionally I would buy essentials for my flat, but never things like new clothes. Trips to London to see my mates were increasingly infrequent, and I would fill the car up to visit my parents less and less too. That frustrated me, and my release was inevitable – I would gamble more to try to dig myself out of a hole.

I was finding it harder to manage my emotional well-being. I felt awful guilt every time I spent all my money as soon as it landed with me – whether through my monthly pay cheque, a big win or even just a birthday present. That guilt came alongside the shame I felt for my social unreliability and all the other things that resulted from my secret life.

My mental health was as damaged as my bank balance – although I would never have admitted that. I didn't really understand the concept of mental health, or that I was truly struggling. The only person I'd really known with mental health issues was Foxy Fowler, my coach at Durham uni who had played cricket for England. He'd gone through many struggles with his mental health, but in the time I was working under him at Durham, he was doing well. After my year group left, he experienced a downturn. I was concerned for Foxy, but I had never seen first-hand the effect it had on him.

I'd no appreciation that my own mental health was becoming a problem. At that time, I still considered mental health a taboo subject. Men weren't expected to talk about their feelings, at least around me they certainly weren't.

My biggest issue was self-esteem. Those around me would have considered me arrogant, full of bravado and thinking the world of myself. Behind closed doors, I increasingly thought I was utterly worthless. I'd gone from being a professional cricketer to a single, debt-ridden gambling addict working in teaching on relatively low wages. I looked at the salary I would have been on if I'd stayed in London and compared my situation with the stage of life my friends were at. I had a low opinion of myself.

I made sure to keep a very upbeat mood at all times for those around me. I wasn't depressed, because I didn't have a constant low mood. But I did experience massive highs and lows, which were directly linked to my gambling. I thought of myself as someone with a gambling habit riding those waves. But really my addiction was a mental health issue already manifesting itself in other ways. There were times when I would get myself thousands of pounds up, but not be able to walk away from another bet. Before I knew it, I'd frittered it all away. And that would leave me feeling utterly bereft, with so much internal anger.

Really, all my arrogance served to do was make me believe I was immune from mental health issues. I couldn't possibly be mentally unwell. That couldn't happen to people like me – even though it so clearly could.

I'd been in Oxford for three years. The first had been broadly good, but the next two had seen huge growth in my addiction. It had resulted in bigger debts (by this stage, they were probably about £30,000, before taking into account my student loan and what I owed my parents) and my mental health had massively deteriorated. As I suffered on in silence, life felt like a daily struggle, becoming ever more challenging. But nothing major had gone wrong (yet) and apart from a few quiet but insistent requests for cash, no one suspected a thing.

Over the next year, that would all change.

7

October 2014

From late 2014, my lifestyle and behaviour began to catch up with me, deepening my gambling addiction further. In October, half a term into my fourth year at the school, I was lucky enough to be invited on a school trip of a lifetime to Tokyo, on a Japanese exchange programme. We travelled to an unbelievable city that was like nowhere else I'd been and, to top it off, the kids were billeted with local families while the staff stayed in a hotel, so I was free to explore the city at night. The opportunity wasn't wasted.

At the weekend we'd visit famous landmarks and beautiful places, but in the week the kids were in school every day, then off to their host families in the evening. We would come into school for early starts, but that didn't stop me having a lot of fun in the evening. That led to some horrendous hangovers and a severe lack of sleep. I wasn't going to be much use observing Japanese lessons even when firing on all cylinders. And I certainly wasn't firing on all cylinders.

In the evening we would head out with our Japanese hosts, who absolutely loved drinking, but would burn out early and head home. My colleague and I would charge on. A couple of times I was out until 3 or 4 a.m. in Roppongi, which had fast become my favourite part of town.

While in Japan, my gambling took a backseat, for a few reasons. First, I was very busy, with so much to see and do. I felt so detached from my life at home that temptation was low. I was just in a totally different place – literally and figuratively. Second, I'm not sure the mate I was with had ever placed a bet in his life, which was a natural deterrent. And third, accessing my gambling accounts was difficult. I found a way a couple of times to make a few bets, but some apps and websites were geo-blocked.

Towards the end of the trip, however, I got a nasty surprise, which sent me into tailspin. While observing an enthusiastic Japanese teacher demonstrate a daring experiment in the kids' chemistry class, my phone was going mad in my pocket. I nipped out of the room to discover a series of missed calls and a torrent of angry messages from someone back home, who had learned something relating to my personal life that I desperately didn't want anyone to discover, regarding a previous relationship.

The thought of this ruined the remainder of what had been an amazing trip. I battled to avoid telling my colleague, and managed to keep it to myself. I felt like staying in Tokyo, not for a couple more days, but for a couple more years. The journey home was unbearable, with my anxiety through the roof. I knew I was returning to face a situation in which I felt I was the villain, the one entirely in the wrong.

I'd no option but to face the music when I returned home, and tackle it head-on. The situation was complex but my ultimate goal was for as few people as possible to be aware of it. I managed that, but it did complicate life in Oxford.

My response to all this stress was inevitable. More than ever before, I gambled. When I wasn't working, I was in my flat or the bookies. Gambling (and, to a lesser extent, alcohol) was the only thing that made me forget about everything else, and escape. Naturally, it only deepened the problem.

My mental health deteriorated further, and I experienced depression for the first time. I felt exhausted by guilt and regret. The sense of self-loathing I'd experienced before deepened, and became more permanent.

The troubles brought on by this situation outweighed a positive in my life. A couple of months earlier, I'd started going out with a colleague. Things had been going well and I actually thought – for the first time since I'd been dumped after uni – that I was entering into a relationship that had a future. She'd joined the school straight out of uni and was bit younger than me. I'd first met her when she was going out with a guy I played cricket with. Before long I'd replaced him, which caused a bit of a stir at the cricket club. There was also some crossover with another woman I'd been seeing for a couple of months. I certainly never made things simple for myself. If I sound like I'm trying to present myself as a bit of a lothario, I really wasn't: I was just a mess.

On my return from Tokyo, I had no choice but to be honest with her about what had happened. This was the right thing to do, but it made our relationship more complicated.

Because we were colleagues, my new girlfriend and I had tried to keep our relationship quiet at first. We would see each other every day at work, and she would come to stay a couple of times a week. The nature of our jobs meant we didn't have huge amounts of spare time to spend together.

Being single had helped me maintain the double life I increasingly led. But it naturally became harder now I was in a relationship. Nevertheless, I found hiding my gambling from her easier than I anticipated and, as always, pushed the boundaries to their limit. She knew I liked the occasional bet but had no sense of the extent.

The Tokyo incident proved to be a catalyst for a huge amount of regret about the way I had conducted myself over the previous couple of years. I withdrew into my shell, and developed serious social anxiety for fear of making further mistakes and upsetting people. I found Oxford a difficult place to be.

I had a lot of great friends in the city, and obviously family close by as well. As I became increasingly distant my sister was quick to recognise that something wasn't right. She had no idea of the extent to what I was hiding.

Eventually, I cracked, and told her what was going on in my personal life. She was her usual supportive self, listening and giving advice, while also being discreet, respecting the confidential nature of my problem.

As my gambling became worse, I leant on her ever more for emotional support. I would go round to her and her husband's flat (which was also at the school) and just burst into tears at any mention of whether I was coping.

Even though the situation was challenging, it wasn't as bad as I was making out to my sister. My real issue was that I was consumed by addiction. What had happened when I came back from Tokyo was the perfect smokescreen; I could blame everything on that but nothing about the real problem in my life. Because of my gambling and my debts, I needed to cry and open up – for just about the first time ever. But I didn't ever really tell her why. There was only really so much my poor sister could do.

The colleague with whom I shared an office also recognised that there was an issue because there were significant changes in my demeanour and behaviour. He had been my line manager in my early time at the school and remained something of a mentor, with whom I was close.

As 2015 rolled round, I was increasingly self-destructive. I was prepared to ditch things I'd once cherished to fund my gambling – and cricket was first. By now I was in my late twenties and, as mentioned earlier, I should have been striving to play for Oxfordshire in Minor Counties cricket (the level below the 18 first-class counties). As it was, I was only really playing club cricket because I liked the guys I played with.

I'd also been qualifying to be a playing member of the MCC since 2010. To get through the probation period, you had to play 10 qualifying games in two years, which I'd done straight after leaving university. So when I got into the MCC in 2012, I was overcome with pride and really enjoyed being a member – even if I'd behaved poorly when invited to go on that tour to Hong Kong. Membership meant I could go to Lord's to watch England in the summer, and I'd had some great days there (which also included some gambling and a lot of drinking). To keep up my membership, though, I needed to play a further 15 games over the next five years. I'd been pulling out of those games regularly, making some awful excuses when I could easily have played.

The MCC's annual subs – which were about £400 if you were my age and didn't live in London – were due on 1 January each year. In 2015, I was broke, and just stopped paying. I thought it was something I could get away with and just catch up on the arrears when that inevitable big win arrived. A year after I stopped paying, I started receiving written warnings from the MCC, who eventually revoked my membership. I just frittered away something that once mattered so much to me.

While playing club cricket for Horspath, I needed to gamble much more urgently than I had before. I was still quick to leave the field at the tea break so I could check my phone but now I even batted recklessly so that I wasn't out in the middle for too long and could get back to my bets as quickly as possible. The result of my own match and my own performance had become less important than the matches I was betting on.

In April 2015 I was due to travel to Cape Town for a mate's wedding. He was a teacher at another school so the wedding, at which I was going to know lots of the guests, fell neatly in the Easter holidays, and I'd been looking forward to it for months.

I was strapped for cash but I'd bought myself a flight a few months earlier after a decent win. I planned to fund the rest of the trip – and much more – with winnings from Cheltenham in March. I wasn't able to make the annual pilgrimage to the races myself – you can't claim you're going on a close mate's stag do every year – and was experiencing all the usual lows that came with FOMO, more now than ever, because of my issues in Oxford and my financial black hole. All the friends I usually went with had taken days off work, and I was stuck at school.

In the racing world, it was a big deal that the hugely popular pairing of trainer Willie Mullins and jockey Ruby Walsh were putting four horses into four races, all as big favourites, on the Tuesday, the opening day of the festival. Lots of people backed all four, including my mates. I wasn't going to miss out either, and put on my usual complicated web of bets, from four-folds to singles. With so many people backing these horses, the bookmakers were watching from behind the sofa.

Everything was going swimmingly when Douvan and Un De Sceaux won their races comfortably, then Faugheen romped home in the Champion Hurdle. Mullins and Walsh's last horse to run was Annie Power, who until the final hurdle absolutely dominated. Unchallenged, she fell at the last hurdle, with another horse trained by Mullins – Glens Melody – pinching the win. It was still a record-breaking day for Mullins.

This was an extraordinary afternoon of racing. The betting industry's immediate estimates were that Annie Power's fall had saved them having to pay out £50m. A Ladbrokes spokesperson was quoted in the papers as saying, 'We've dodged the most expensive bullet we've ever faced and the god of bookmaking moves in mysterious ways.'

Well, that bullet hit me where it hurt. I had so many bets on that I stood to win £50,000. I'd watched the race alone in my flat, having finished a sports session with the kids and then running back to make it in time. Annie Power was so far ahead and in such control that I was actually celebrating the victory before the final hurdle had been crossed.

When she fell, my reaction was genuine disbelief and complete despondency. I had not won a penny and panicked massively about not being able to afford the trip to South Africa, and rued all the things I could have done with the rest of the money, not least all the debts I could have paid off. I couldn't stop thinking about it. I won't pretend that there wasn't some consolation in so many other people being in the same boat.

I dusted myself off and looked ahead to the next day's racing and attempted to win the money back. It didn't work. Soon enough I was on the phone to a mate who was also going to the wedding, asking for a significant loan. Thanks to him I made it to South Africa.

Coincidentally, my girlfriend was also heading to South Africa at the same time, but we had arranged to go independently – even before we had met. I was off to the wedding while she was due to stay with a former gap-year student with whom she was close. As things were going pretty well in our relationship, I decided – despite my financial situation – to make a proper holiday of it, and to spend some time with her before linking up with all my friends who were coming out for the wedding.

For much of the first week, the two of us did standard touristy things in my favourite city in the world, Cape Town. We were very kindly put up by the parents of this former gap-year student in their lovely home, which had an annex, where we slept.

On one day that week, I'd arranged to meet some of the others who had arrived early for the wedding. My girlfriend also had plans with her friends, and so we spent the night separately before reconvening the following day to head to Simon's Town, down the coast.

That day I played golf at the stunning Clovelly Golf Club in Fish Hoek with the groom and two other mates. We followed a great game with beers in the sunshine, then – having left our golf clubs in one of the guys' hotel rooms – headed to Camps Bay for a boozy lunch at Paranga, a superb restaurant with stunning sea views. More people, including the friend I would be staying over with, joined us as day became night and we kicked on to the famous Le Caprice bar. I spent the next few hours getting smashed, dancing badly and catching up with some old friends who were now living back home in Cape Town.

At about midnight, my race was run and I decided to head home, but the mate I was due to stay with still had plenty left in the tank. So I decided to head back to stay with my girlfriend. It seemed like a sensible enough idea, except that my phone had run out of power. I'd been using Uber to get around because it was cheaper and safer than a standard cab. The obvious solution would have been to ask a friend to order me an Uber but I didn't want people to know I was sneaking off. So I chose to wander along the Camps Bay beachfront to pick up a taxi – something I'd been expressly advised not to do while in South Africa. But after who knows how much to drink, I didn't really care whose car I was getting into.

I found a cab rank and got into the first car. I only knew the street name and suburb, not the exact house, but backed myself to recognise the house. I told the driver this, then got into the front seat and promptly passed out, fast asleep. Who knows how long later, I came to in shocking fashion. While I'd been out cold, the driver had veered off the road and crashed the car into an oak tree on one of Cape Town's tree-lined avenues.

A passer-by had called the emergency services and they had arrived quickly. I woke to blue lights flashing and the sound of police and paramedics getting to work on the car. It was mayhem. I was shaken, dazed and confused, but could tell there was blood all over the dashboard and what remained of the windscreen. I looked to my right, and the driver lay slumped and motionless. It was immediately clear that he was dead.

I felt as if I'd sobered up, but clearly I hadn't. I was absolutely terrified and my instinct was to escape. The paramedics were trying to resuscitate the driver but also wanted to attend to me as I was covered in blood, dazed and limping badly as I got out of the car. My right knee was in searing pain. Still drunk, I repeatedly told them that I wanted to be at home with people I knew. I desperately didn't want to be whisked off to a local hospital without anyone knowing where I was and no way of contacting them.

The crash had drawn a number of onlookers. One of them approached me and told me he could get me home. Of course, I should never have agreed, but I did. He could have taken me anywhere, and this constituted not cooperating with the authorities. But I just wanted to escape the awful nightmare.

Fortunately for me, he was as good as his word. He got me to the right street and then we spent some time trying to work out which was the right house. We got the right one but I think the father of the gap student thought he was being robbed. When he opened the door to see me standing there, he was in a state of total shock. So was I. I was covered in blood, holding my shoulder and neck, which were throbbing, and by now barely able to stand. To make things worse, I couldn't even explain what had happened to me. He woke his wife, who went and grabbed my girlfriend. She was concerned, but more than anything I don't think anyone could understand what was going on.

They whisked me off to a private hospital, where I was checked over. They removed glass from various parts of my body, and I had some tests. I kept being told just how lucky I was. It must have been 4 or 5 a.m. by the time I was discharged with lots of medication, and a pair of crutches, and told to come back the next day for further examination, including X-rays. Remarkably, beyond severe whiplash, knee ligament damage and some cuts and bruises, physically I was fundamentally fine. The death of the driver and my own near-death experience would leave some much deeper mental scars, though.

I woke the next day in turmoil. I was in pain, but also felt severe guilt about having fled a crime scene, and feared the consequences. I couldn't stop thinking about the driver, and wondered what it all meant for his family. I decided to go to a police station. Before we returned to the hospital, I got in the car with the mother of the family I was staying with, and we retraced an obvious route back to Camps Bay. Remarkably, we found the scene of the accident – the car had been removed, but there was glass and debris left on the street.

We arrived at the nearest police station. I walked in and explained what had happened. There was no computer system, just a massive black logbook that had record of the incident. I gave a voluntary statement and that was about it. I asked about the driver's family, but they said there was no record of him or his family. The cab, it appeared, was unlicensed. The woman I was with explained that there are so many road accidents in South Africa that this sort of tragic occurrence wasn't unusual. I was devastated but didn't know what else I could do except report my involvement.

We returned to the hospital, where I was prescribed more medication and rest. After a long night's sleep in the annex, and an apologetic and embarrassed departure, my girlfriend and I headed for Simon's Town – where the iconic penguins live at Boulder's Beach – as planned. We spent a few days there resting (both of us) and recovering (just me) in very low-key fashion. I was extremely anxious about what had happened, and what would happen next, including the financial implications because the family we were staying with had paid all my medical bills because I couldn't afford to. My parents stepped in and paid them back in the following days to avoid making them wait until my insurance payout arrived.

I should obviously have just gone home to Oxford. My mum was so worried about me she even considered flying out. Instead, I stuck to the plan and said goodbye to my girlfriend, joining up with the wedding party at a friend's villa. Ignoring all medical advice, I got absolutely battered at a party a couple of nights before the wedding. Probably down to a combination of medication and my own recklessness, I was so drunk that friends considered calling an ambulance once more.

The following day was the stag do, then the wedding was the day after that. Needless to say, I didn't just have a couple of quiet nights in. My face was grazed and bruised, and I had a limp, but I still didn't slow down. This was a dangerous form of escapism – I was also gambling a lot, whenever I was alone – and people couldn't believe what had happened, or how quickly I'd 'recovered'. But I had not come close to processing what had happened. I felt I needed to make the most of being alive and threw myself into the week in every way.

So the wedding was on a Thursday, followed by a big after-party on the Friday. On Saturday morning I was on a flight back to Heathrow. It was, by some distance, the worst flight of my life, and I was sick most of the way home. I landed late on Saturday, wallowed in self-pity on Sunday and was back to school for a pre-term staff meeting the following day. All this meant that I returned to work having not got to grips at all with what was an extremely traumatic event.

The weeks that followed were extraordinary and I visibly struggled. I could hardly have wished for more support. Mum and Dad were very concerned about my welfare and the school – especially the headmaster's wife, who was in charge of safeguarding – couldn't have been more supportive. If I needed time off work, it was there. If I needed counselling, they would arrange it.

I pushed all that away. With my life falling apart even before I was involved in a crash that claimed the life of another man, the last thing I wanted to do was expose myself to an expert who might be able to see through my web of lies. Everyone knew what had happened to me but I didn't want undue attention. Missing days of school was guaranteed to put me in the spotlight, so I just kept going, keeping an even lower profile than I had before the break.

I constantly trivialised what had happened to me, and tried not to dwell on it. I felt I already had enough to worry about. Frankly, my horrific experience in South Africa seemed to pale in comparison to everything else that was going on day to day, managing everything that came with my addiction. But I couldn't escape the crash. I regularly woke up screaming, with flashbacks punctuating horrible nightmares. My girlfriend, who had obviously been through it all with me, became used to this. The act of sleeping – I had been asleep when the accident took place – led directly to images of the horror I had woken up to in the crashed cab.

I spent many of my waking hours anxiously wondering what had actually happened. Was it a pure accident? Was the driver looking at or talking on his phone? Was he drunk, or on drugs? Could he even have done it on purpose? It wasn't that I was bitter or callous, it was that I had no answers to a huge event in my life. I couldn't take a taxi for a long time afterwards. And if I could avoid it, I wouldn't sit in the passenger seat of a car.

For the first time, I had some very dark thoughts. I wondered if it would have been simpler if I'd died in that crash instead of, or as well as, the driver. I'd got myself into a horrible mess with the gambling, but no one knew about it. Perhaps dying in a car crash would have been the easiest solution to my problems. Perhaps then people would have had sympathy for my death, rather than having to deal with it being 'self-inflicted'.

But I also used it to my advantage. I leant on my sister ever more, knowing that she would dutifully feed back to my anxious parents that the accident had had a profound impact on me, quietly enabling me to further bury my gambling issues.

As I attempted to fund my ever-escalating gambling, my debts rose – because I exploited the support available to me. I was extremely fortunate with how I'd been looked after by everyone after the crash. The family we had stayed with were incredible, rushing me to a private hospital and then funding the care I received because I wasn't in a position to do so. Because my concerned parents had stepped in and paid them back immediately while we waited for the insurance payout to land, which obviously took some time, I was very lucky not to be financially out of pocket at any stage of the painful experience. But I was still struggling financially, having cycled through all the well-known payday lenders, having exhausted all reasonable requests at the bank of Mum and Dad, having taken that loan from a mate after the Cheltenham shocker, and having maxed out my overdraft.

So I needed other ways of funding a gambling addiction I couldn't control. It's a measure of the level of care provided by the school that when I went to the bursar asking for a loan to help me out, they agreed. I was to pay it back through deductions to my salary over the following months, which would give me even less money to gamble with – good – but less money to pay off my other mounting debts – bad.

But even that wasn't enough. The loan from my mate before South Africa had opened my eyes to a new funding route. And the accident meant I was now the subject of pity. I began asking friends – particularly those who I had been in South Africa with, or those who weren't connected to school – for loans. I would blatantly lie, explaining that I'd had to pay for treatment and was waiting on the insurance.

By that summer, I'd been given five or six significant loans – all between one and two thousand pounds each – from people I knew. I was very specific about who I asked, targeting those who I thought had the means and would oblige. Frankly, I was shameless and opportunistic.

I asked people I knew in London, but always those slightly removed from my direct friendship groups. Having sat out the early part of the cricket season after the accident, I played for my old school in the Cricketer Cup, a competition for the old boys of various public schools. After a game against another school, I was chatting to one of their players, who told me he ran a hedge fund, so clearly did pretty well for himself. We got on well and exchanged numbers. A week later, I asked him if he could help me out, telling him my well-honed sob story, and he agreed.

I'd borrowed off individual people before. But this was different. Before, it was small, manageable amounts from people I knew well and was therefore under pressure to repay. But I was now making targeted approaches to wealthy people further from my immediate circle – and for much more money. As before, this was bad news for the outstanding payday loans and their accruing interest, as I still concentrated on repaying the money that came from people I knew, rather than faceless institutions. This might have been an emotionally simpler approach, but it was financially punishing.

I kept my head down at school, and through the summer holidays. I ran a couple of my cricket coaching courses, which were extremely lucrative and kept some much-needed cash coming in.

Returning to school in September for the new school year, my fifth in Oxford, I found my personal situation even more difficult. Feeling low, my gambling worsened, and my physical health deteriorated in a way it never had before. I was by now massively overweight and totally despondent. I thought almost constantly about the car crash, except for when I gambled.

I decided that this simply had to be my final year at the school – and I was offered an easy escape route. An old family friend, who I'd known since I was a kid, was a headmaster of another school, which wasn't too far away and had a great reputation. I had the utmost respect for him both personally and professionally, and I'd always liked the idea of working for him as we were already close. From the circuit, I also knew some of his staff.

Earlier in the year, before I went to South Africa, this headmaster had sounded me out for a job. Someone I knew who coached all sports, but particularly cricket, as well as being a key member of the teaching staff, was leaving, and the headmaster wanted me to be a like-for-like replacement for him. I was by now a qualified teacher, with four years under my belt, and a good reputation at the school. Obviously he – like everyone else – knew nothing of what was going on behind the scenes in my life.

I seriously considered the offer, but hadn't really thought of leaving Oxford before. So I told my current school about the opportunity, and they responded by offering me a significant promotion – an indication that for all the chaos behind the scenes, I was still doing plenty right. The flattery and a bit of extra money were enough to convince me to stay. I had to make the decision before the Easter holidays because of the terms of my notice period, but with everything that went on in South Africa, I lost sight of the issue for a few months.

By the autumn, though, it was very much back on my agenda. I was severely regretting my decision to stay, so I contacted the headmaster again, in confidence, and asked whether there would be any scope for a move ahead of the next academic year, in September. I explained that I was ready to leave, and it didn't need to be exactly the same excellent job he'd offered me earlier in the year (which by now had obviously been filled), and that I was prepared to wait patiently in the ranks for the right thing to come up.

He asked for a bit of time to consider his staff roster but soon got back to me and offered me a position at the start of the next academic year. This was great news. Change was something I feared but it was also something unavoidable now. My ever-deepening double-life meant I just had to leave the school before I got found out.

By October half-term, in 2015, my financial situation had disintegrated even further. In my search for money I'd been deceitful again. I was well-regarded at my cricket club, where I'd been the first notable 'signing', and was considered an asset in a period of success. I used this to my advantage, asking for a loan from the club who, despite limited funds, agreed to my request.

It was agreed that I would pay the loan back in instalments over the following 18-month period. I gambled the loan itself away quickly but was determined to keep up with the repayments. Having borrowed on all sorts of different fronts, I probably had £50,000-worth of gambling debt by now.

All the teachers were tired by the time the holidays arrived – teaching is an exhausting job and at a boarding school many of us had responsibilities seven days a week, often late into the evening. But I was really on my knees. I was working extremely hard but I was also living my other secret life, and the effort required to keep them separate and the school side of things afloat was hard to bear.

To almost everyone around school, I was something akin to a model teacher. Kids liked me because I was young, nice to them and not scary like some older members of staff. It also helped that I was heavily involved in their sporting endeavours, which provided them with an escape from their classrooms. I was great with the parents, especially those who came to watch their kids play sport. We would chat on the touchline, and I'd come to know some of them very well.

To my colleagues, I was a reliable figure too. Having grown up in similar schools and watched my parents pour so much into their jobs, working hard was no issue for me. It was what you did. If I was asked to run an extra sports fixture because someone else couldn't, the answer was 'yes'. If I was asked to go on a school trip, the answer was 'yes'. I was generous with my time with the kids – if they wanted extra support in the classroom or on the sports field, I wanted to help. The worse things became behind the scenes, the more I put into life at school. Only a few people knew that there was another life behind the mask.

When the holidays arrived, I tended to crash on the sofa and splurge on the stakes. I could finally let my guard down, and stop acting. I no longer had to keep up a pretence. I could breathe but, as before, I lost lots of money. It was made worse when I had little to do, as was the case with this half-term. I couldn't play cricket because the season was over, or much golf because the weather was closing in. It was a long enough break to do something big – I'd been to Kenya with mates in 2013, then had the Japan trip in 2014 – but now I couldn't afford to do much other than stay in Oxford and head to my parents for a couple of days. Even though I didn't have much money I just sat at home and burned through the little I had left.

It was perfectly normal for me to run out of money before the end of the month. Indeed, the last few days before payday were the only times I would ever cut my cloth, lowering stakes and opting for accumulators, rather than the bigger, simpler bets that I would make when I had access to more cash. But during this month, October, I hit rock bottom with weeks to go. In November, that lead to an act of deceit that was new to me.

That month, I grew a moustache, with some other members of staff, for 'Movember'. I was normally clean shaven and pretty well kept (bar my ever-growing waistline) but I grew a ginger handlebar moustache that made me look ridiculous. It was a good laugh, and all in the name of charity. Or not.

I should have just set up an online donation page but instead I simply pinned an envelope to the notice board above the photocopier in the corridor outside the staff room. I emailed all staff informing them – and then reminding them a few days later – that I was raising money, and said the same to any parent I came across, too. My relative popularity meant the envelope soon had plenty of cash in it, so I emptied it and took the money back to my flat for safe keeping.

It was a recipe for disaster. If I had access to cash, I'd gamble with it. Within a few days – with payments to make to banks and individuals – my salary was largely gone and the £5 and £10 notes I'd been donated were all I had. I couldn't resist taking it all to a betting shop (a place I'd almost stopped visiting) day after day and, inevitably, losing it. I felt horrendous, but there was plenty of November left to run, and I planned to simply win the money back so I could make a big donation online for the amount I'd been given – and more.

Of course, that win never came and all that money intended for men's mental health charities was gambled away – and no one knew. I had never intended to steal the money and use it for gambling, I was simply unable to control myself. I felt sick then, and I feel sick recalling it now. Gambling had completely changed me.

8

January 2016

By 2016, my addiction had taken full control of me.

My financial situation was a mess and getting worse, and I was going to increasingly desperate lengths to obtain funds as I continued to spend wildly beyond my means. Gambling consumed my thoughts and monopolised my time. The time between each bet was shortening, to the extent that it was now the first thing I thought about in the morning and the last thing I did at night. I slept less and less. My mental health was increasingly dire. I was a serial liar. I was terrified of being exposed. I'd lost control in every respect.

But I now went to another level entirely. Money would become truly worthless, just a means to bet. I became numb to my wins and losses. The number of gambling accounts I owned increased as much as the bookies would allow me. I thought ever more about my next bet. And that thinking time reduced, because my next bet arrived ever sooner.

I started the year by confronting the fact that I was changing jobs. Over Christmas 2015, I'd experienced the fear of returning to school like never before. Even if I knew I had a way out lined up, the seven months that still lay between me and my departure were extremely daunting. I feared my secret life and past mistakes would be exposed.

So I decided I could no longer pretend that everything was fine. I knew it was time to move on, and wanted to leave with as little fuss as possible. I arranged to meet a member of the senior management team and explained that the time was right for me to resign. I mentioned that I had personal issues and that I was unhappy in Oxford, but omitted the biggest issue of all: that I was a raging gambling addict. They agreed that I should leave the school for my own sake. A difficult conversation with the headmaster followed, but he agreed I should go too.

When it was revealed to everyone else that I was leaving, the response was mixed. My parents were excited for me. They were glad that I was going to work with their old friend and at a school they admired. They knew I'd had some issues – although I'd mostly managed to keep from them what these actually were – and felt that a change would do me good.

And after 30 years in the teaching industry themselves, they also recognised that I'd reached a stage in my career that suited a move. They had seen plenty of male teachers arrive as enthusiastic newcomers only to become part of the furniture, often remaining bachelors, without ever considering a move. Teachers are creatures of habit, and schools such as the one I was at can be comfortable environments. I'd been teaching for five years, and a move would provide a fresh new challenge as I approached the end of my 20s.

But others – teachers, parents and pupils at the school – were more confused. I was in only my first year as Head of Year, which was an excellent job for a teacher my age. I was also Head of Cricket, another very good role. Everyone assumed things were going swimmingly, and I was often asked why I was leaving. I would bungle a slightly unconvincing excuse about it being a great opportunity at a good time in life for a change.

My mind was permanently filled with guilt – about my gambling, my debts, all the lies I was telling, and about the fact that nothing I now did was authentic or genuine. I was addicted to lying as well as gambling – I was a compulsive liar as well as a compulsive gambler. Telling the truth actually became difficult, because it endangered the many lies I already had in place. One lie would compound another, and keeping it all secret is, it turns out, addictive, too. In many ways, that was the greatest challenge and pressure I felt.

In my final months at the school, I experienced another form of guilt; I knew that I was moving – or at least joining my new school – for all the wrong reasons. I was seen as an excellent teacher and a 'good signing' for the school, when in fact I was a total liability, and knew it. I'd gone through job interviews – with people I knew and respected – keeping this all under wraps. It was all a facade. The disconnect between who others thought I was and who I knew myself to be weighed heavily. I was constantly performing.

My chief focus was on getting out of the school unscathed, which I did. As far as I know, no one else found out about the double life I was leading. That was a huge relief. I was particularly glad to make it away without damaging my sister and her husband's reputation. They had worked hard to settle into their own life there and the last thing any of us needed were problems that undermined that.

There's a fair bit of pomp and ceremony at the end of an academic year at most schools, and this one was no different. The school and its staff do their best to shower their departing colleagues with praise and presents. I did my utmost to keep my head down throughout.

They held an official leavers' event, and any teacher who had been at the school for six years automatically had a speech made about them. Generally, teachers loved this, but I was delighted to have only been there five years, thus avoiding the spotlight too much. On the Monday after term ended there was an annual fancy dress party for staff. I spent the whole day getting drunk, keeping the lowest profile possible and desperate for it to end. My colleagues had done a whip-round to get me a gift. They thought I would appreciate a cheque; I was very grateful, but gambled it away in minutes, tossing it aside without consideration.

When that was all over, a summer holiday that was damaging in almost every way began. Leaving the school brought about one of the most harmful changes in mindset of my gambling journey. I felt that I'd made it out alive and that I'd dodged a lot of bullets in the process. I felt relieved, and I saw everyone I knew from that time in a different light. That included the parents of the kids I'd taught. The relationship between teachers and parents at schools like this is extraordinary, and I used it to my advantage almost as soon as I left.

Parents at private schools spend a lot of money on their kids' education, and want to be engaged and present in that process. At the school I taught at, they would come to watch sports matches I coached, and we would chat on the touchline and conduct a post-match analysis as the kids ate afterwards. I also had responsibilities looking after the kids in the boarding house, which left me *in loco parentis* and as the point of contact around sensitive issues like homesickness. As a tutor to a number of kids, my role was to champion them in the school – which meant parents were always keen to keep me onside – and, again, I was their point of contact.

Having also been on a number of school trips with parents, I'd built a strong rapport with many. On those trips, they had watched me be the responsible adult while on duty in the daytime, then a fun dining and drinking buddy in the evening. There were fundraising dinners where I'd spent the evening with them, and cricket matches between the fathers and sons that I'd set up. As a younger member of staff, I was perhaps more approachable and, throughout my time at the school, had had fewer issues with parents than many of my colleagues. I can honestly say that I considered many of these people friends.

Having exhausted what seemed like every other avenue to fund my gambling, and safely out of the school, it didn't take me long to start approaching these parents for money, too. I'd learned a bit about them – including what they did for a living – and knew how much the school fees were. I knew that these were people who – when viewed through a purely financial prism – could afford to lend me a sum in the low four-figures. They usually obliged, although they must have thought it very odd to be approached in this way.

When I contacted them (generally via email), I lied, as I always did, about why I needed the money. The normal excuses were that 1) I had a tax bill to pay, due to a benefit-in-kind associated with moving school and being given accommodation; 2) paying back fees associated with my teacher training (which the school had funded) because I was leaving the school too soon; 3) the cost of moving house and setting up a new home. All three were utterly made up, of course.

I knew that what I was doing was wrong but I was so far gone that this was a boundary I was prepared to cross. The only other option seemed to be stealing, or committing fraud of some kind. As ever, I set out with the best of intentions to pay the money back.

In the course of the summer, my girlfriend and I split up but this didn't rock me like other relationship breakdowns had. It made sense to go our separate ways as she was also leaving the school to move to London.

In truth, I don't think it was a desperate wrench for either of us to part. I was secretly quite happy to be single again, because it made my double life easier and meant I didn't have to manage a long-distance relationship while making a fresh start in a new place. I felt guilty that she didn't know who I really was, adding to my deep self-loathing. Far from blaming her for the break-up, I knew where the fault really lay.

I filled my time in inevitable fashion.

I went on a holiday with mates to Hvar in Croatia, which provided a neat encapsulation of the struggles I was experiencing. My ever-changing financial situation meant that even securing my place on this holiday was a saga. I was going with mates from uni who had stayed in London when I left and were now operating at a different financial level to me. They were booking, and asked me to commit. On that day, I'd lost a large chunk of money so I said I couldn't. I prevaricated for as long as I could until they issued an ultimatum: was I in or out? By chance, I'd won big that very day, so was able to book.

It was a nice feeling to be going on holiday. When the mate who organised it all told me that we didn't have to pay for the hotel until we checked out, it was a mixed blessing. It meant I would have more cash to play with in the short term, but also meant that I could be back in financial strife by the time the holiday actually came round.

This am-I-in-am-I-out build-up to the holiday was emblematic of most of my social activities. I was reliably unreliable, committing to things when I'd won money, then withdrawing when I didn't. As it happened, I did make it to the holiday but I very nearly didn't make it to the end. These boys enjoyed the finer things in life and, frankly, I couldn't keep up.

One afternoon, one of them decided we should go out on a boat, so went to do some research. We expected him to return to consult with us, not book a private speedboat with a driver. It all sounded superb, but my heart sank when I heard the price. I could barely have afforded a wooden raft, let alone a private speedboat. But it was too late – it was booked, and I was far too proud to admit that this was a disaster waiting to happen, not least because there were still many more days of merriment to pay for.

Unsurprisingly, my anxiety was compounded by a hangover of epic proportions (in fact, I spent most of the week pissed or hungover). The fear was deep; could this be the moment that I'm rumbled by mates? I had a couple of hours to spare before the boat trip, and spent them sweating under a parasol, relentlessly emailing friends, parents from school, and any other contact I knew asking for money – and fast. By now, just a few weeks after I'd first done it, this seemed like totally normal behaviour to me. Desperate times were calling for desperate measures. Could any of them save me from what felt like a full-blown crisis?

Remarkably, someone got back to me, wiring the money immediately. I had blamed the financial pressures of moving school and house, and insisted that I would be able to repay this in full as soon as I returned to school and received my first salary payment.

I was able to enjoy our afternoon on the boat, and an entertaining evening too. West Ham were playing, and one of the boys was a lifelong fan, so we tuned in after dinner. He also liked a punt (while having no idea what I was up to at this time), and encouraged us all to lump on Michail Antonio to score the first goal.

When he did, we all won big and celebrated wildly, long into the night. For me, though, it just added to my tiring facade. They had no idea the stress I'd been through that day, the lies I'd told, or just how much it meant to me that Antonio had popped up at the back post to score. It was good news – spectacular news! – that he'd scored, but the weight of the lies and the deceit were mounting by the day, and I could barely manage. If this kind of behaviour happened once in a while, it would be exhausting. I was now doing it on a daily basis.

By the end of the holiday, I felt at a low ebb. The Antonio win meant that I'd been able to pay for the hotel, but I'd received a series of painful reminders of my predicament. I'd spent most of the week pissed, with my guard down. I was in the company of some of my best friends. Yet I still couldn't open up to them about my issues and went to increasingly desperate measures to avoid being rumbled. They would probably have been supportive, and could have helped, both emotionally and financially. I was just not brave enough to reach out. I wondered whether this was because I was simply too scared, or a sign that I was now beyond help.

As I moved schools, I left the cricket club in Horspath – and sadly, things had really soured. I'd taken the loan from the club in 2015, and had also been lent money by an old boy who was a supporter of the club, as well as one of my teammates.

As usual, I began by keeping up with my repayments, but eventually couldn't manage, so quietly stopped paying. I left the club on the grounds that it was too far for me to travel to play every Saturday, which wasn't an unreasonable reason to leave, especially as my new school weren't prepared to give me time off to play. I'd been increasingly flaky that summer, first because I had an injury, then because my mind was elsewhere and I couldn't be bothered.

The trouble was that my departure coincided with ceasing to pay my creditors back, and sympathy from the club for my issues dried up. I believed that the three separate loans were all secret but, as so often in a small environment, there were several people who knew what was going on. Bridges were burned, and I betrayed people who had given me so much support. As summer became winter – and I was now living a little further away – I was being chased for repayments, but I just ignored them every time they got in touch.

At certain times, I had the money to make repayments for loans like this. There were times when I was thousands of pounds up. But I would never pay off more than the bare minimum. There are reasons for this. First, my sheer greed. Second, my desperation to place my next bet meant I needed to keep the cash for myself, and not 'waste' any money on repayments. That is how warped my mind was.

But I also had other payback priorities. By now, I'd borrowed money from so many people that I couldn't even remember some of them. While I was organised in other aspects of my life, and a diligent file-keeper at work, I just hadn't drawn up a document to keep track of my financial situation. Seeing it all in front of me would have been overwhelming.

My priority in terms of repayments was the payday loans, which accrued interest at alarming rates. The loans I'd had from individuals were generally interest-free and I could either lie my way to deferring them, or just lay low. Because I did it all so much, it was becoming normal to me.

My relationship with the bookmakers changed that summer, too, as my need to gamble became greater. It was a love-hate relationship – they were causing me so much trouble, but I couldn't live without them.

Anyone can get a free bet. Since the advent of online gambling – and with it, casual gamblers getting involved more often – freebies have been used by bookies to lure in new customers, with adverts in the *Racing Post*, online and in the tabloids, especially around the biggest events in the horse racing calendar. I'd certainly enjoyed my fair share over the years; indeed a few years earlier, on the train to Cheltenham, I'd systematically opened 22 new accounts with different bookmakers, lumping the free bets all in one direction – and I won! The bookies won too, because those accounts were now open, and I kept using them. And boy, did I use them.

By the summer of 2016, as a big spender, I was lavished with privileges by the bookies. These came in many different forms: free bets, offers of hospitality at big sporting events, and even a personal 'VIP account manager' – a direct contact at the bookmaker for all my gambling needs.

Just as I'd been in the early days, I was an absolute sucker for these free bets. Despite my love of live sport, free things and being well looked after, I was less interested in the invitations to the big events. Those seemed to me to be a route to exposure – I didn't want to go if other attendees knew that I'd only been invited because I was a massive gambler. And I didn't want to tell people I knew that I was going as a guest of a bookmaker because that would have been a big red flag, too. So I would turn these incredible opportunities down, but ask my VIP manager if I could have more free bets instead.

Each bookie had a different system for their VIP managers, but generally, I would email or text them, only calling when I wanted to kick up a real fuss.

And making a real fuss wasn't that rare for me, as I tried to leverage my gambling spending to get more and more from them. I would run out of money as I waited for paydays or my next loan, so I would contact my VIP manager, asking for free bets, and reminding them how much I'd spent that month, or telling them that another bookie was being particularly generous and I was thinking about gambling exclusively with them, threatening to close all my other accounts.

With some bookies, I was on loyalty bonuses, meaning that I would receive a free bet at the end of the month based on a certain percentage of what I'd spent. If I ran out of money on, say, the 20th of the month, I'd contact them, demanding I receive it sooner. I would even try to tug on their heartstrings, telling them I was in strife. My status as a heavy gambler was a bargaining chip that I used and abused as regularly as possible.

As I became more desperate, I was increasingly aggressive with them. Generally, they were very obliging, despite my rudeness. And little wonder. They made huge profits, and I was a huge contributor. Anything they gave me for free would be back with them before too long.

*　　*　　*

Of course, by now it was clear that no geographical move could stop me gambling, as I'd hoped when I had originally switched from London to Oxford. Sure, I thought that some of my issues would evaporate: I associated Oxford with the Cape Town crash, so hoped leaving would ease that. And the environment was one in which I simply was not happy. To move on from these sources of anxiety was very welcome.

The new school seemed a perfect fit for me. It wasn't too far from where my brother and sister remained in Oxford. I knew various members of staff already, including the headmaster and his family. Loving sport seemed to be a prerequisite, and there was a healthy social culture among the staff, which you can probably guess I was looking forward to. The school was all boys, meaning the sports I ran took centre stage, and it had a slightly less stringent timetable; there was still Saturday school, but no duties on Sunday. I was really looking forward to moving.

I officially made the move to my new school at the start of August, in the middle of the summer holidays. When I arrived in my small flat, there was no one else around that I knew, and wouldn't be for a few weeks while they all enjoyed their holidays. Besides a week away with my family and the odd trip to see mates here and there, I was basically alone, gambling, for a month until I started work. I vaguely hoped the new term would at least disrupt the flow of my gambling, denying me time on my phone.

When term did begin after what felt like an eternity, something wasn't right though, and I really struggled to settle. As I'd expected, the people were great and the school environment was a great fit. The trouble was, I was now only a fringe player.

The headmaster had been clear with me about my initial supporting role, with responsibility only increasing as other staff left and jobs opened up. I had just assumed it would be a bit more demanding from the start. Without being cocky, compared to what I was used to (working manically to manage a series of responsibilities in the classroom and on the sports field), this was a doddle. I spent a couple of hours in the afternoon coaching sport, and taught some cover lessons. But that was just about it.

My colleagues, meanwhile, were working a full tilt, yet I felt like I'd nothing to do. I tried to tread the fine line between being helpful and getting in the way; often, that meant quietly slipping back to my flat, turning on the TV, and gambling relentlessly on sport. At the weekend, I had school sports fixtures on a Saturday, but – unlike in Oxford – I would then be off until Monday morning, leaving Sunday free. That meant I gambled and got drunk.

All this made September 2016 a rollercoaster month. I was gambling far more than I'd ever been able to while at my old school. I had some extraordinary wins, and found myself making a staggering amount of money. At one stage, I calculated that across my many online gambling accounts I had more than £96,000. I enjoyed a ridiculous hot streak gambling on golf, backing Rory McIlroy heavily. I would back players at the start of the tournament, then back them even more heavily once it began; this was a tactic that either worked brilliantly or disastrously. In racing, I would put on double and treble bets on well-fancied horses with short odds, and huge stakes. When I won, I would reinvest the winnings in a similar fashion.

But still, it was never enough. I kept going, and ended up losing it all. None of my winnings ever made it into my bank account, the idea that this was real money just didn't exist in my mind.

One obvious issue was my greed, but I also had my own idiosyncrasies and whims. I wanted £96,000 to be £100,000, in part because I'd developed a strange obsession with round numbers. I remember as I added up all the money, every account bar one had a nice, clean round number; so I chased wins from that one account that was out of step and, of course, things began to fall apart.

In my mind, I kidded myself that when I got to the milestone of the next big round number, I would take the money and walk away, paying off my debts as I went. Of course, I wouldn't have done that. As I lost it, it didn't feel like I was losing almost £100,000, a truly life-changing sum for a man with big debts and no possessions of greater value than a set of golf clubs. The constant desire for more was evident in my belief that while having almost £100,000 would solve many issues for me, it wouldn't fix everything. I never had enough. A million wouldn't have been enough.

With the money spread across multiple accounts – even when I had £96,000 in total, I probably didn't have more than about £4,000 in any single account – it didn't feel like I was suffering disastrous losses in the moment. Until, that is, I had lost it all. The money had flowed through my fingers. Although it's scarcely believable, it took just a couple of days to lose it all. And that had always been the way; it took time to build things up but it could all disappear in a flash. And it wasn't until it was all gone that it would dawn on me what was happening, that I was losing something very real. I was devastated.

October and November 2016 were some of the most challenging weeks of my life as things unravelled. It started when my pay cheque arrived at the end of September and, for the first time ever, I gambled it all away in a single day. More than £2,000 came and went. I'd been wasteful before, but never like this.

As a result, the only funds I had access to were possible winnings, or further loans. Desperate, I wasn't shy of asking for money, as I demonstrated one night in the local pub in the village. It had not taken me long to become a regular there, along with a number of my new colleagues. Another regular was a bloke who drove a flashy car and wasn't afraid of letting people know he wasn't short of cash; it was a badly kept secret that he was the local drug dealer. Unlike in my London days, I wasn't terribly interested in his wares and I barely knew him, but I enjoyed having a chat with him when pissed, and he was always friendly enough. On this occasion, when pretty well-oiled – and my guard was down – I asked if he would ever be able to lend me cash. There and then, he took a load of £20 notes out of his wallet and started counting them out for me.

The next morning, I woke up – hungover – and could scarcely believe what I'd done. Borrowing from a stranger, who I knew mixed in suspect circles? Clearly, I was prepared to ask anyone for money now. Paying money back was rather more difficult, but I prioritised him, knowing that I could get myself in trouble if I didn't. I escaped unscathed and managed to give him his cash back, but the danger wasn't lost on me.

It was another round of borrowing that brought my troubles even closer to home. The summer before my move, I'd reached out to the colleague I'd shared an office with at my old school. He was my superior at school, but had always provided wise advice and had become something of a confidante for life in and out of school. I'd opened up to him, without ever revealing anything about my gambling. Had he known, I have no doubt he would have informed the school. I trusted him, and he looked out for me. I asked for a loan of £1,000, and he agreed.

I promised to pay it back in September, and did, after a big win on the horses in that mad month. After pissing my salary away in a day, though, he was one of the first people I turned to for help. While coaching kids at a rugby tournament, I'd suffered a big loss gambling on my phone and a matter of days after paying him back the first loan, I was asking for the same amount again.

Again, he agreed, although a little more suspiciously and reluctantly this time. And again, I was able to promptly pay him back, thanks to a big win. But the vicious cycle continued and, when I lost big again (after an even shorter period), I was messaging him straight away.

This, coupled with the fact that he'd heard some worrying rumours about me approaching parents for money at the school he still worked at (and wielded increased authority in) meant that he'd heard enough. My sister and her husband were colleagues of his, but he decided to contact my parents. He didn't know them well, but had met them a couple of times, knew they were involved in the teaching world and would share his concerns.

As it happened, they had been increasingly worried about my situation, too. For the first time in a while, I'd recently asked them for money. They knew I was emotionally all over the place and had their suspicions that it was down to more than just the upheaval that came with moving schools. When my old colleague told them about my borrowing, and given that they knew I'd liked the occasional punt in the past, they started to wonder if the issue was gambling.

This all happened in the week after a hugely damaging half-term break during which I'd spent an inordinate amount of time in London casinos, and getting drunk. All the indications were that I'd become an alcoholic, too. I would drink to combat guilt, shame or loss (including the loss of money, which was regular). I would put away can after can of Stella Artois, and my weight ballooned further because I'd barely done any exercise for months.

This school holiday also showed how I'd lost all sense of money's value. I was gambling huge amounts, obviously. But I'd completely stopped spending money on essential items. I didn't buy clothes and, even though I desperately needed to, I wouldn't pay to go to the dentist because I considered it too expensive. What I would spend my money on, though, was an Uber for the hour journey back from London, even though I'd a return train ticket.

One weekend at the start of November, my parents travelled from Sussex to visit me – giving me no choice but to talk to them. The three of us sat round the small table in my new flat, which I'd done very little to make feel like a home. At first, I resisted their attempts to get me to open up. I said I couldn't tell them. I was ashamed, embarrassed and very scared. But Mum particularly made it clear that they were going nowhere until I provided an explanation. She told me that they thought gambling was the issue, and wouldn't take no for an answer.

The three of us were soon in tears as I owned up – to an extent. I said that since moving from Oxford, I'd struggled, and had been on a gambling binge, quickly racking up debts of around £20,000.

They were shocked and very upset. Both were supportive, as they always had been. Mum, I could tell, just couldn't take being worried sick about me any more. Dad was cross and confused, but desperately wanted to help. And what I'd told him meant that they could help. They weren't happy, but left later on when we had all calmed down, promising to provide any support they could. As parents, they were in uncharted territory, with their 29-year-old son opening up about his issues – like I said, to an extent.

Early the following week, Dad got in touch. He'd taken some financial advice, and arranged to take out a bank loan that he would then loan to me to help pay off the debts I'd told him about. He asked me to inform him how much I owed each individual, and he would transfer me that exact amount. He then wanted me to send the money on, providing him with evidence that I'd done so.

They were trying to treat me like an adult, but I didn't deserve that privilege. I'd already lied to them, merely revealing the tip of the iceberg, and my response to receiving the money showed that I needed far more help with my addiction than just being offered support. I didn't follow his instructions. As ever, I paid some of the money back, providing proof from my online banking statements that I'd done so. For others, though, I fabricated evidence, doctoring images so that my dad thought the job was done. He'd gone to huge, costly lengths to help me out of trouble. In return, I lied to him, then gambled the rest of the money away. He'd had the best of intentions, but really their loan simply enabled me.

In the following weeks, I was understandably on edge. It was important to me to project an image to my parents that I was doing better. They had no idea how deep my issues were, because I didn't let them in. My parents wanted to know everything I was up to, but I kept them at an arm's length. My mum was really struggling with the revelations and was having trouble sleeping. I knew that she wanted to hear reassuring noises that things were improving, but I was wary about talking to them too much, or giving too much away. The colleague from my old school was brilliant, talking to them and me, all while being totally discreet. But it changed my relationship with him, and I looked to keep my distance from him, too. I was angry with him, feeling like he had gone behind my back, even though I should have been grateful.

My mum made me have some counselling. To appease her, I met a mental health counsellor a few times in a nearby town, and she was lovely. But I wasn't the most willing participant, and she said little that resonated with me, and didn't seem to have great understanding of addiction, or gambling. I would listen, but there was no connection there. Before too long, I stopped going and again lied about it to my parents.

All these new lies, and the total abuse of my parents' generosity (of money and of spirit) sent me deeper into despair. I'd managed to open up to them just enough, alerting them to some issues, providing some answers that quietened a few of their questions, while also allowing myself to continue gambling. The fact is, I didn't yet want to stop, or be fully rumbled. This was hardly an effective long-term strategy, but my thinking was increasingly hand to mouth – or hand to phone. I just thought about my next bet, which was now akin to a heroin addict's next hit.

9

December 2016

One Friday in December 2016, my life changed – in a very big and very unexpected way. Since my break-up with my girlfriend, I'd been messing around on dating apps like Tinder and Bumble in the many hours of the day that I spent on my phone.

I'd been on a couple of dates and had a bit of fun, but I was quite certain that I didn't want, and couldn't manage, a relationship. I was hiding too much from too many people already, so the last thing I needed was another person with a keen interest in what I was up to (although a shoulder to cry on wouldn't have gone amiss). I was a mess, and knew it. And I was begging, borrowing and pretty much stealing to prop myself up, so couldn't contemplate even occasionally offering to treat someone else. It just seemed like a non-starter.

So it was fitting, perhaps, that I stumbled into a relationship when I really was least expecting it, and on one of the more remarkable days of my life. That Friday I had two appointments in Oxford. The first was back at my old school where, ominously, I'd been summoned by the headmaster for a 'chat' – which didn't sound like it could possibly be good news.

The second was a happier meeting. The week before, while back in Oxford visiting my sister and her family, I'd matched on the dating app, Bumble, with a woman called Charlotte. She was also a teacher and we had spent the whole week getting on famously, messaging each other on the app. I'd enjoyed our chats and, given that I was coming back to Oxford anyway, I thought 'why not?' A nice afternoon with a nice person might cheer up a troubled bloke.

But I had to get the tricky bit out of the way first – the meeting with the headmaster. He was adamant that this should take place at his house nearby, not in his office at the school.

Unsurprisingly, I was hungover, as it was the first day of the Christmas holidays and the staff at my new school had celebrated the night before. This added to my anxiety about the unknown nature of this meeting. I declined his offer of a drink, not least because I wanted to get out as quickly as possible. This was no time for hair of the dog.

He didn't mess about with much small talk, informing me that he'd been made aware by several parents and a school governor that I'd been approaching them for money.

I didn't deny it. He informed me that what I'd done wasn't breaking the law but he hoped I knew what I was getting myself into, and that I was doing so with good reason. He told me to be very careful, given the small world teachers in such schools lived in. I'd not moved far away, my sister and husband were still teaching at the school, and my parents and brother were in the industry too. Get this wrong, he said, and it could damage everyone I cared about.

This was a message I should have welcomed. It was sound advice, and came from a good place – especially as he kindly promised to keep it confidential. I made enough 'right noises' to ensure that he wouldn't tell my parents, who he knew, about the situation. That was good enough for me. My greatest fear was that all of this would get back to them. I lied that my parents were very aware of my financial situation, that they knew I had money troubles. Of course, they didn't know the extent of my problems and as far as I was concerned, it would be staying that way.

I listened to what I was being told but didn't really take it on board. The hangover didn't help, but I just wanted the meeting to end and the only bits of information that really hit home were the 'positive' aspects: that what I'd done wasn't illegal, that my parents wouldn't find out, and that he wasn't reading me the riot act. I should have left that meeting very concerned. Instead, I was relieved. I had no real regard for my reputation at a school I'd worked at for five years and had only left a matter of months before. My thinking was massively blurred and naive, and I paid no heed to anything but the next few hours.

As it had happened, the next few hours were a lot of fun. I had a quick bite of lunch with my sister and niece (who had been born the previous year), and strolled into Jericho, a part of town I knew well, to meet Charlotte. We had agreed to meet for a wander round the city centre and get a coffee, which suited me down to the ground. I knew it wouldn't cost me much and, if it went disastrously, wouldn't take long. It didn't go disastrously at all.

Charlotte:

Patrick and I experienced a whirlwind start. After a week of messaging, we enjoyed a pretty normal first date on a Friday afternoon. The connection was instant, and talking was as simple as it had been by message. We had been back and forth almost constantly for a week since matching with each other.

I have no idea what made me swipe right to show my interest in him, because he wasn't normally what I would have gone for. But it was instantly clear we had a lot in common. We both taught in independent schools, and were very family-orientated.

When we met, one thing that struck me early on was that the whole event really seemed to matter to him. He seemed kind, genuine, interested and definitely charming – but he also clearly wasn't in it for just one thing, like a lot of guys.

It was like we'd known each other for ages. I felt very at ease in his company and was a little giddy and nervous, because I knew I was enjoying myself.

The date came to a natural conclusion and he walked me home. As we were on the short walk back through Oxford, he held my hand, which I thought was quite quick, but on my doorstep, we shared a little kiss, too. When it was all over, he said 'thank you', which seemed a slightly strange reaction, so I asked why. And he just said 'thank you for spending time with me'. It was weird, but sweet. And I was thankful to spend time with him, too.

The non-stop messaging continued and we were soon on a second date, this one in the evening. We had a drink, then a Chinese at a favourite old haunt of his in North Oxford. He ended up staying for two nights! Everything was going well.

Over the Christmas holidays, we stayed in very close contact, writing these long essays to each other over WhatsApp, which I daren't look back on as they'll make me cringe. It felt like we were telling each other everything, and really opening up. Around Christmas itself, we had done some long video calls and were becoming more connected by the day.

Everything moved rapidly, but it didn't feel wrong. He seemed straightforward and just lovely. Sure, he was clearly impulsive and liked doing things in a hurry – it only took him a couple of weeks to tell me he loved me, which again seemed quick, but I know I was thinking the same thing. I just had not plucked up the courage to say it. By the time we both went back to school, I'd met his family and things were going very well.

By the second date I felt that I'd met the woman I would spend the rest of my life with. I wouldn't have pursued it seriously if I really didn't. Everything just felt right. Everything, that is, except me. I still had my many issues.

The period over Christmas when the two of us messaged non-stop and I had the near-constant butterflies that come with a special new relationship actually helped my gambling a little bit. I was at my family home and my mind was occupied by Charlotte. I was telling my family all about her, and the lift in my spirits was obvious. I still gambled – of course I did – but perhaps not with such all-consuming aggression.

Charlotte was switched on, almost intimidatingly bright. She was attractive, and I couldn't believe my luck. It didn't take me long to fear losing her and that made the thousands of lies that were part of my backstory so problematic. I was as honest with her as I felt I could be.

I opened up about previous relationships (including my failings) and the reasons I'd left jobs in London and Oxford. What I did hold back was the depth of my financial issues, and anything about gambling. I didn't talk to anyone else about my gambling, so it seemed obvious to keep it from her, too. It was my secret. In the early days, it didn't really come up. Over time, my love of sport meant she knew I liked the occasional innocent flutter, but I gave her no reason to think anything more of it.

For the first six months, being in a relationship was simple enough. She lived in Oxford, I was at school, 40-odd miles away. One of us would drive to the other's place for a night in the week, getting up early to do the return journey before work started. And we would see each other every weekend, often on Sunday as I had work commitments on Saturdays. We saw as much of each other as we feasibly could, and things continued to progress as quickly as time would allow.

It meant I was only ever hiding my addiction for a day or a night at a time. I would give her the fullest attention I could, and worked hard at this. Before meeting up, I would stack bets on to tide me over, then check them when I got a quiet moment alone, or as soon as we weren't together. I slept badly, so would often get my fix at night as she lay next to me.

It also meant I could hide that I was an alcoholic. I'd always drunk a lot but in the first couple of months after moving schools,

I went to another level. Charlotte, by contrast, has never been a big drinker. She likes a couple of glasses of wine or prosecco every now and again, and has a bit of a passion for gin. Some of our evenings together involved alcohol, but not all of them. When we were apart, it wasn't unusual for me to finish work, then put six Stellas away in two hours. That could be pints in the pub, when I could afford it, or those comically large pint-sized cans elsewhere when I was hard up. The culture among my colleagues meant that I wasn't often drinking alone, but I would occasionally.

I would ensure that I got my fill of booze when not with Charlotte, so I could be somewhere near my best when we were together. I'd been living a double life before we met, but I was entering a new, even more self-destructive phase.

The relationship had very quickly become very important to me and I kept my guard up vigilantly. I always made sure that I had enough money to get through our time together, often by borrowing from anyone who would lend to me. I would gently manipulate our plans based on what my financial situation was at any given time; it helped that she wasn't lavish in her spending and, being in a similar job, wasn't overly flush for cash either. We liked doing simple things together and generally didn't have expensive tastes, although both of us were fond of a lovely meal out when possible. So whenever I'd a bit of spare cash – after a win, or after borrowing – I would make a point of treating us to something a bit special at a restaurant.

There were a couple of events that brought us closer together. During the Easter holidays in 2017, we went skiing together, something we both enjoyed, but had not done together before. It had been the same old drill for me, booking the trip after a win, then nervously trying to ensure I could hold onto enough cash to pay for it all. We cut every corner we could financially, and there were moments when I was budgeting like crazy to make sure I stayed afloat. I had nowhere to hide at all – it was only the two of us on the trip – and time by myself for gambling was hard to come by. But it was a wonderful holiday that bound us even closer together.

The other moment that brought us closer together came a few months before, in February, when it had become public knowledge that the headmaster of the school at which I worked – who was also one of our closest family friends – was extremely ill with cancer. My family had known for a little while that he wasn't well, and that the prognosis was bad, but I'd been given very few details because of my position as a staff member.

During the February half-term, as the newly appointed Master in Charge of Cricket, I was to lead a group of 15 boys and their parents on a school cricket tour to Cape Town (returning to the scene of the crash that still haunted me, two years on). While I was apprehensive about returning to Cape Town, and the inevitable surfacing of bad memories, it was also a place I'd had a lot of good times and knew well. I could never erase that moment from my mind, I was no longer experiencing flashbacks and thinking about it with such regularity. It also provided me with an opportunity to catch up with people who had been very good to me in the past. I'd been looking forward to it for months and it was shaping up to be the best school trip I'd ever been on (and I'd been on a few by now) – not least because the attending teachers didn't have to contribute financially.

The headmaster was also due to travel on the trip, which combined his three greatest passions: cricket, his school and people. But, not long before half-term, he took me to one side and said that he would not be travelling as he needed to stay at home for medical visits. He was disappointed, but took the news in his stride and remained outwardly sunny, because that was how he approached life. For everyone who knew him, this was devastating news.

We went to Cape Town and a talented group of kids pulled off some amazing results. The headmaster was on our minds and there did appear to be a determination to make the trip a success in his honour. He was extremely proud of our results. I was proud of what the boys had achieved, but overcome by sadness at what was going on at home.

At the end of the spring term, it became clear that he would be unable to continue working as he underwent emergency treatment. He would be replaced temporarily by one of his deputies. Before too long, that temporary measure became permanent. I would never see him in a professional capacity again.

I found all this desperately difficult to deal with. I considered him to be a second father figure and not only was I close to him, his wife and three children, but I felt so sorry that they had to deal with private anguish very publicly.

Some months later, he died. I was grateful that I had had the opportunity to tell him how much he meant to me, and thank him for his support – in and out of school. I felt guilty that he'd had no sense of what was really going on behind my eyes, and behind his back.

From my own perspective, I'd settled in after my rough start at the school and had a bit more responsibility, which I enjoyed. My professional and personal lives had both felt on the up – but the headmaster's death affected me badly. Like the car crash in Cape Town and the various relationship trials and tribulations over the years, I was left feeling confused and bereft. As ever, I responded by suppressing my emotions and gambling more.

At school, his departure changed things. It had been so sudden and tragic, and he was such a central figure, that everyone – staff, pupils and parents – seemed in a state of shock. His involvement at the school had always meant that I'd respected my job, not least because I didn't want to compromise a relationship that felt so important to me. Now that we had lost him, my professional enthusiasm dwindled and I worried less about making errors. I was gambling a lot, and was probably less concerned about being caught.

Alongside all this I felt guilt for starting a relationship where I wasn't the man Charlotte thought I was. I was working hard to keep my hidden life from her. There were times when we were going for dinner at 7.30 p.m. and I still hadn't received the money I needed at 7. That was highly stressful, and not sustainable. I suppose my attitude towards the relationship became emblematic of my wider approach to my addiction: I'm surely going to get found out at some stage, so I might as well enjoy this beautiful thing I have stumbled into.

And it was beautiful. Without Charlotte, things would have been even worse. Thanks to the joy she brought me (which was also a distraction from the incessant need to gamble) and the support she provided through a troubled time, I didn't feel alone, which perhaps limited the damage of my addiction, despite its silent acceleration.

We had only known each other a couple of months, but Charlotte was a pillar of emotional support. The headmaster's death was a desperately tough, drawn-out process that comprised shock, sadness and grief. She'd only met the man I was grieving for on a couple of occasions and obviously didn't know him well, but appreciated how close we were and helped me manage the distress. I dread to think what would have happened at this time if it wasn't for her.

Charlotte:

In the early months we were together, Patrick and I moved fast, knew we were experiencing something special and spoke lots, but were only seeing each other a couple of times each week around our jobs. I would stay over in his bachelor pad at the school (for a bloke of his age who liked a drink and worked pretty hard, it wasn't as messy as you might think), and he would travel up to Oxford.

He was sociable, popular and, frankly, more straightforward than most people I knew. Of course, there were little quirks and he wasn't perfect, but there wasn't anything particularly out of the ordinary. We all have our little issues.

We had similar jobs and seemed to be in a similar boat financially. I didn't think it was strange that he might ask those very close to him, like me, for a bit of money; I'd borrowed small amounts from my parents before, too. I lent him a bit of cash a couple of times when he said he was stretched towards the end of the month, and he helped tide me over on occasions too. He was never tight, there were times when we ate well and it suited me that we were one of those couples where it wasn't weird for the girl to take the guy out for dinner – not just the other way round. There wasn't anything lavish about our lifestyle, but I felt content and looked after. I certainly wasn't nagging him for dinner at The Ritz. I just wanted to spend quality time with him.

He was open to discussing his emotions with me, which I thought was great because so many men I knew weren't. And it seemed less unusual as I got to know his family – who I got on brilliantly with immediately – better. They were very outwardly emotional people.

The first time I met them, he cried when saying goodbye, but so did they. I thought it was slightly odd as I didn't do that when saying goodbye to my parents, and had never seen it before, but also found it sweet that they were this close. He struggled with goodbyes generally, which perhaps had its roots in his time at boarding school, when goodbyes would last quite a while at an age when he wasn't ready for them to.

There was evidence of some anxiety and he struggled to sleep. But there wasn't anything that desperately affected our relationship; I slept like a dream, so had no real idea what he was up to while lying next to me. He implied I helped him manage his anxiety, which he also played down.

One thing I did learn pretty promptly was that his phone was … his. It wasn't mine to go near, and he was extremely *secretive with it. I'm not sure I ever even touched it – just to pass to him, or answer a call. He always had it as close to his person as possible, and it was normally in his hand. A couple of times I woke from my deep sleeps to find the light of his phone illuminating the bedroom. I would ask what he was up to and he'd say he was reading articles about sport or WhatsApping friends. We would watch TV, and he would be glued to his phone, only half paying attention to the programme.*

This did bug me from early on, but it didn't feel unusual enough to raise seriously. I tutted a few times, making clear that I'd rather he gave me his full attention at that moment in time, rather than his iPhone. But he was someone who always wanted to be up to date, whether that was with what I was up to at any moment, or with the sports that he followed so avidly.

The other thing was that he was a keen user of the bathroom. When he went to the loo, he would really take his time – and always took his phone. I almost wondered whether he had some digestion issues. And he would enjoy a lengthy bath more than any adult I knew. The door would always be locked behind him, which I didn't like given it was only ever us in the house and I sometimes wanted to wander in to interrupt his bath for a chat! But I respected his right to a bit of alone time, and accepted it as part of his method for managing life.

I worked extremely hard to be at my best around Charlotte, which was made simpler by the manageable periods of time we spent together. I'd spent the entire half-term break in Cape Town, then the skiing holiday at Easter meant we didn't spend day after day in each other's company at home, doing normal things outside term time for a little while. I was financially vigilant and smothered my gambling habit so that she wouldn't know.

My phone was my blind spot. I knew my use of it annoyed her, but I was now as addicted to using it as I was to gambling. I felt that if someone got on my phone, everything would be exposed. Keeping my phone close was a long-running habit, right back to when I'd been devious in relationships at uni and particularly when I first had a smartphone in the City of London. In the few months before I met Charlotte, my phone use had escalated again – at least in part because I'd been playing around on the dating apps.

From early in our relationship, she would tell me to get off my phone. I would try, really hard. But a minute later, I would have picked it back up, and she would rightly have a proper pop at me. It really was the only thing we ever argued about.

My reaction could be irrational, because my behaviour was too; I wished I could articulate how much I wanted to pick it up. She couldn't understand how anything could be that important that I needed to give it so much attention.

I could move it into another room, but even when it was out of sight it was never out of mind. I would physically shake thinking about the possibilities it held. Often, even when I'd no cause to go on it, I would simply unlock the phone as a reflex. Once the phone was unlocked, I would begin exploring again – normally on a betting app.

On my phone I'd carefully curated folders to keep my secret safe from anyone just shooting the handset a passing glance. In those folders lay around 30 gambling apps for every bookmaker you've ever heard of, all the social media apps, so I could gather tips and information, as well as sports' broadcasting apps, so I could watch the action on the go. On top of that, my WhatsApps and emails – there were perhaps five email accounts – were on there, detailing all of my contact with parents from my old school and more. It was my little handheld hub for gambling. It was the key to my secret life.

So I was very jumpy about it. I was physically compelled to hold it and the thought of anyone else touching it filled me with dread. If I received a funny WhatsApp pic that I wanted to show her (or anyone else), I wouldn't pass the phone over. I would take it over to her, and flash the screen at her. If I was on the phone to someone and they wanted a word with Charlotte, I would do anything to avoid handing the phone over, like putting it on speakerphone, so it remained in my control. If I felt someone was looking over my shoulder at what I was up to, I would become shifty, or snap at them to go away.

Conversely, I'd developed a strong hatred of my phone's fundamental job: to make calls. Perhaps this also had its roots in my boarding school upbringing, with calls a reminder of the distance from loved ones and homesickness. But I'd also come to associate it with tough conversations that you can't escape from. Perhaps it was also just my anxieties speaking and I was pre-empting issues. I feel there's a generational divide with phone calls. For people my parents' age, calls are the default mode of communication – they're no-nonsense and they're direct. For younger people, messaging is more comfortable. That's certainly true in my family. I preferred to let my parents' calls ring out, then message them back 10 seconds later. If my phone flashed up saying I had a voicemail from anyone, I would be filled with dread.

I was very good at finding excuses for being on my phone. It helped that it coincided with a time when many people spent time glued to their phone, and excessive screen time wasn't the hot topic it is now. Many people my age were on their phones constantly and we 'needed' our phones for work matters (although the amount I used mine was beyond the pale and clearly contravened official policy; I was on it so much that I couldn't just be sending work emails). My phone (over)use had always frustrated my parents, and it was a long-running joke in my family (which made me conscious of it, so I worked hard on my behaviour) but over the years even they were using theirs ever more. My excuses were pretty easy to manufacture. At home, I was messaging mates, scrolling social media or reading about sport. If I was at school, I was firing off work emails or checking my diary.

My use of my phone while at my previous school had been managed and disciplined. I'd learnt to live without it while I did my job. Now, at my new school, that had changed dramatically. Perhaps the quiet period after I first moved there contributed, because I spent my whole life on my phone then. So when my calendar got busier, I couldn't put the thing down.

* * *

By now, I could barely get through a lesson without placing a bet. At times, I would plan classes so that I could guarantee a few minutes sat at my computer with my screen out of sight as the kids beavered away. Horse racing takes place in the afternoon; my lessons after lunch were increasingly farcical. I would bet on my phone while coaching kids on the sports field, too.

I was barely 30, but my prime as a teacher was behind me. In those days, my lessons had been inventive and interactive, and I paid attention to every child at every moment possible. I was proud that I was continuing the family business in teaching and helping to shape bright young lives.

As hard as it was for me to recognise then and admit now, the pupils ceased to be my priority as my gambling gripped me further. I would sit them down with a task and tell them to get on with it, while I sat in front of them on my computer. When they needed help, I would go and attend to them in my own time, with little urgency. Colleagues noticed this occasionally but I was cunning and sly. I never faced any consequences for it, so things slipped even further. If the school had known about my shortcomings and loss of focus, they would have been horrified.

One thing I did have in my favour was that I retained a great relationship with the kids I taught. They liked me, liked being taught and coached by me, and we had a natural rapport because I was able to create a relaxed, but respectful atmosphere. That filtered back to the parents, who I was also getting on well with. Since Christmas, I'd had a bit more responsibility, but one aspect of my job that I still gave my absolute all to was being the kids' tutor – which meant being directly responsible for their progress and the point of contact with their parents. It was a similar arrangement to my previous school, with some boarders and some day-children.

My new colleagues noticed my strong relationship with the kids, too, and that I never shirked extra hours, taking on after-school clubs, sports fixtures and duties. I was happy doing all that, as long as I had access to my phone to gamble, and I understood the optics of my role.

It was in the company of my phone that I generally filled the hours during which I couldn't sleep. It helped that Charlotte and I were generally only staying together a couple of nights a week because, while I slept badly in her company, I was much worse when alone. At least when she lay next to me I was worried about the bright screen waking her up and dialled back my usage a bit.

When we were together, I would at least turn off the notifications that alerted me to all sorts of aspects of the sports I was gambling on. I would go to bed each night, but I honestly would barely sleep. I'd lie there, betting on my phone, and sometimes watching on my iPad. Strangely, by now, this was pretty much the only time I settled in to watch sport. Even as a lifelong lover of all sports, I wasn't really that interested in consuming the action – I only cared about whether I'd won or lost my bet, and what that meant for my next bet. A brilliant goal or delivery left me unmoved. What got me excited was a win, for me.

Not being able to sleep deeply frustrated me, increasing my angst and self-loathing. When I was alone at night I would put bets on – and the time of day meant I wasn't gambling on things happening in a similar timezone, so my knowledge of my subject was significantly reduced – then lie there until a little buzz on the phone told me what had happened. If I did manage half an hour's sleep, I would wake with a start and check my phone.

The lack of sleep, of course, was also inextricably linked to my relentless drinking. I'd often try to drink myself to sleep so I'd get eight hours of cherished shut-eye. I might get the uninterrupted sleep, but it was low-quality, and I'd have an awful hangover the next day, reducing my productivity and lowering my mood.

I'd forgotten how it felt to be fresh, and not be groggy, hungover and generally run down. I was in a state of constant exhaustion and, when I was tired, I would make more poor decisions that would contribute further to my misery. I ate terribly, stocking up heavily on the ample school food available, starting with a full English breakfast every morning. I was a very big bloke – heavier than I had ever been at almost 17½ stone (110kg), which was about four stone (25kg) more than I weighed when I was a cricketer. People commented, especially the other sportier teachers who would rib me about how much I ate. That did nothing for my plummeting self-esteem, but I didn't make any lifestyle changes to reverse the situation. My family noticed my steady weight gain, too, but were not especially worried because my relationship with Charlotte was making me happier around them.

And it was brilliant, of course. Being with Charlotte gave me something to crow about, and a positive topic of conversation. Everyone saw me as a much happier person. But, in some respects, it was also brilliant for keeping my gambling addiction a secret – since other people saw I was happy with her, they asked me fewer questions. I leaned on the support of my mum, sister and other confidantes less. I met up with friends less because I was with her at weekends, and those friends didn't feel like there was much to worry about. Had they seen more of me, they might have realised that there was.

Less than six months after we first met, we decided it was time to move in together and I asked the school if I could move into a flat in the village that the school had use of, so that Charlotte and I could live together (and she wouldn't have to live in a flat in a boarding house in a boys' school). I asked for this to happen from the summer holidays onwards. The school agreed this was a positive step.

On the surface, it made perfect sense. We were smitten, and we weren't seeing as much of each other as we would have liked. Charlotte was paying rent in Oxford, which prevented her from being able to save for a deposit for a house. If it had been a case of us paying to rent somewhere roughly halfway between our schools, I simply wouldn't have been able to afford it. My accommodation was free so it seemed logical – and helpful – for her to move in, even if her daily commute was pretty hefty.

It had happened more quickly than either of us perhaps expected, but this was very exciting, and I did want to do it. It was a natural step, albeit a big one so soon in our relationship. It also filled me with anxiety and apprehension, because I knew I would have so much more to juggle and hide.

10

March 2017

I had three lives. There was my family and relationships – my personal life. There was my job – my professional life. And there was the most demanding of the lot – my gambling life.

For many years, I'd been able to keep them separate. But over time, they had grown closer and closer together. My gambling affected every aspect of my behaviour and was banging on my door, threatening to expose itself to everyone I knew.

Clearly, Charlotte moving in would make concealing my gambling much harder. But between the decision to move and the move itself I'd made a series of serious mistakes, and started sailing much closer to the wind.

My gambling addiction got involved in my life even when I wasn't gambling. My behaviour was driven by addiction. As a compulsive gambler, I was also a compulsive liar – about any topic going, big or small. My addiction made me angrier. My financial situation now had a reach that was way out of my control, affecting so many people. My addiction needed funding, and my need for money sent my behaviour in all directions.

In March 2017, for perhaps the first time ever, I allowed my gambling addiction to very directly and very negatively affect my teaching – and to the detriment of the kids, who I'd always put first. I was doing plenty wrong around my job to facilitate my gambling, but it generally took place in the shadows. But not this time. This time, it was right before the kids' eyes.

One of my favourite aspects of my job was coaching rugby. In the spring term, that meant taking the U11 rugby sevens team, which we called the Colts. This school had a strong culture and tradition when it came to rugby, and the results this team achieved were a source of great pride. We always had one of the very best sides on the circuit, and it was a privilege to be entrusted with the side in my first year at the school.

It was my job to coach them (which wasn't too tricky, because they were talented boys) but also to ferry them to and from their fixtures and tournaments. This had its positives – the kids and myself were very happy to miss large chunks of the academic day for a bit of sport – but it had its downsides too. These were long days, often in awful weather. And I had to drive the minibus. At this time, I'd normally be the only teacher present, but occasionally I had a colleague on board, too.

Driving the bus was a role that came with the territory of taking a sports team. There were plenty of tests and hoops to jump through to prove you were fit for the job, but I'd done this for years across two schools, so was used to it. But being at the wheel with other people's precious children in the back was a huge responsibility – the sort that's easy to underestimate – and was often very challenging. It's not simple navigating Britain's motorway network while close to a dozen over-exuberant 11-year-olds squabble, question your driving technique, and request you pump up the volume on their favourite tunes. All the while they're subtly trying to stuff their faces with Haribos, loaded sneakily into their bags by their parents and always a recipe for an explosion of energy.

It was Cheltenham Festival week, which automatically meant that my mind was only half on my job as I took the boys to a tournament at a school in north-west London. That morning, I'd heavily backed a well-fancied horse called Neon

Wolf, running in the first race of the day, around lunchtime. Encouraged by some tips, I backed it in a single, but also in a double (two selections that both need to be successful for the bet to win) with Might Bite, who was running later in the day. I'd put a lot of money on this, having had a great start to the week financially. I'd won big on the opening day, Tuesday, with a double that included the superstar horse Altior, and Tiger Roll, who has also since become a household name. I wondered whether Wednesday, and my bets on Neon Wolf, would be the day that would get me out of all the trouble I was in.

At the school rugby tournament, we had two teams competing. One was starting earlier, so went ahead with two of my colleagues. I was due to bring my U11s a little later in a separate minibus.

In a neat coincidence, Neon Wolf's race was at 1.30, which would allow us to arrive at the tournament, check in, get the warm-up underway – and for me to watch the race. I'd also located a car park and picnic spot on the way to break up the journey, so the boys could eat their packed lunches and prepare for the tournament. While the boys noshed away, I could sit in peace and place a load more bets for the afternoon's later races.

My plan was going perfectly. The boys were ready to leave school on time, for once, having remembered to bring their assorted scrum caps, mouth guards and the rest. As we neared my chosen picnic spot, we were slightly delayed by some unforeseen roadworks that caused my anxiety to build. I became racked with fear that my carefully laid plans would be ruined, and I wouldn't be able to place the bets or watch the race. That fear became even deeper when, as I was driving, I spotted a notification on my phone – which was being used as a sat-nav – from a bookmaker. They were offering enhanced odds for a short period of time on Neon Wolf. I was confident Neon Wolf would win, and was desperate to place further bets at these very attractive odds.

The traffic made my blood boil. I needed to make these bets – and then watch the horse storm home. I couldn't afford delays. Eventually, we made it through the traffic, but time was very tight. As we turned off the main road, and the picnic area I'd picked came into view, I had only a couple of minutes to pull up, get the kids out of the minibus and place this bet with the enhanced odds.

But as I approached the car park, I spotted another issue. There was a height-limiting barrier at the entrance to prevent coaches turning up and dumping dozens of people. I didn't have a clue how high my minibus was but made the dangerous assumption that all was well and approached the barrier with next to no caution. There was a sudden bump, and the bus ground to a halt with some alarming scraping sounds coming from above. It was clear that, no, we had not slipped under the barrier with the ease that I'd hoped.

There was instant commotion at the back of the bus, mainly amusement, but also a little discomfort at having been thrown around a bit. Some of the boys were just dumbstruck. One of them helpfully piped up: 'I don't think we can fit under, sir.' That comment made me angry, and the boys seemed surprised because I'd always laughed along with quips like this. But partly out of frustration, partly out of embarrassment, and partly because I was going to miss the chance to place this bet – and perhaps even miss the race on which I'd staked so much – I was hot under the collar.

I tried to reverse out. But we were stuck. Eventually, with a bit of extra throttle, I managed to scrape us out and parked up on the kerb adjacent to the car park. The bus was positioned illegally, but in sight of the picnic spot.

In the previous few minutes, I'd flagrantly ignored every bit of training I'd received on driving the minibus. If any other teacher had seen me do this, they wouldn't have believed my stupidity. The well-being of the kids was my most important job. The school rightly took this very seriously and in that moment I'd let myself down, badly.

The boys filed out, totally silent. I sent them off to eat their lunch and was soon coming over handing out the sweets that I always brought with me for tournaments (and normally used as a sugar rush and edible morale booster between matches).

This time, each sweet was an olive branch disguised as a jelly baby. As ever, they were very well received. Having calmed myself, it was a relief that none of them were hurt – even if some of them were still alarmed. I gathered them round and began the motivational team talk that preceded every tournament. Admittedly it normally took place on the pitch, not in a picnic area, but desperate times called for desperate measures.

I began by apologising, then made a pretty ambitious request that the boys tried to keep what had happened between us, and block it out of their minds. After a chat about the games that lay ahead, they got back on the bus and we completed the rest of the journey to the tournament.

By then, I'd inspected the minibus's roof. It wasn't pretty and had considerable damage. I told the boys, who obviously couldn't see for themselves, that there was nothing to worry about, just a scratch. I'd also got the access to my phone that I craved. I was too late for the enhanced odds bet, but I still stuck a load more bets on, even more than I'd planned to.

I tried to make up for lost time by cutting short the boys' lunch, but by the time I pulled up at the tournament, strategically parking under a big tree with low-hanging branches, the delays meant that we arrived late at the tournament, and I missed the race.

When I wasn't able to watch a race or game I had betted on, I had a strange ritual for finding out if I'd won. The obvious solution would have been to check my online account, where the winnings – or not – would be updated immediately. But I didn't like that. Instead, I would go to the *Racing Post* app, so I could re-read the live blog that they ran.

So that's what I did, as we arrived and unloaded the bus. It's safe to say that my foul mood wasn't lifted when I discovered that Neon Wolf had finished second and that I'd lost another considerable whack of money. I was livid. My mind and stomach were doing cartwheels.

I couldn't afford to let the boys know anything (more) was up. We met the boys' excited parents and my colleagues, one of whom offered to take the warm-up while I checked us in to the tournament. I told him I needed to nip back to the bus for an extra layer. In truth, I was plenty warm enough. I was sweating. What I really needed was five minutes to myself to process the last hour of my life.

I got into the back of the bus in an attempt to avoid the attention of any onlookers, and laid myself across the back seat with my head in my hands in uncontrollable tears. I'd no idea what to do. I'd lost thousands, a sum of money that a Premier League footballer could hardly afford, I'd caused significant damage to school property and I'd let myself down horrendously in front of the kids, who I'd also endangered. Who knows what they were telling their parents right at this moment. I felt truly desperate. For the first time, I felt truly suicidal. That option seemed simpler to me than carrying on like this.

A few minutes passed. I knew that the first game was starting soon and I had to get back to my job. Using some bottled water from a packed lunch, I washed my puffy face and headed back to the playing fields. Remarkably, the boys played superbly that afternoon, outclassing every opponent. I had to say and do very little. The watching parents were gushing in their praise of my coaching style. I smiled, but my mind was elsewhere.

The boys were allowed to go home with their parents after the tournament and, as it happened, all of them did. That left me alone with my minibus. I got in but, before setting off, made sure to shower the evening race card at Wolverhampton with poorly researched bets. Not only had Neon Wolf lost that afternoon, but all my other bets had too. Everything I'd won on the Tuesday was gone.

The hour-long journey seemed to last an eternity. As tears streamed down my face, I considered driving the bus off the road. But I made it back to school and, knowing that the bus would be used for another activity promptly, set about clearing up the boys' mess in the back. As I did so, I felt a wave of violent nausea and was involuntarily sick in a bush behind the bus. Was my body telling my mind it had had enough of this constant stress?

What I should have done was return the bus, and email the Bursar and Head of Sport, informing them that there had been an incident. But I feared the financial implications and wrongly believed I would have to pay for the damage. I also feared this could bring my mental state crashing down. So I went to the staff room, and put the keys away for the next colleague to collect.

By the time I made it to my desk the following morning – very hungover, having spent the evening in the pub trying to numb the pain and guilt – there was already an email from the Bursar, with a subject line quoting the bus's registration plate, the word 'damage', and the previous day's date. I was filled with dread. He knew that he could collar me at assembly (which was compulsory for all staff) that morning, so I decided not to go.

I'd actually had dealings with the Bursar and HR from the week I arrived at the school six months earlier, back in September 2016. I was in disarray at that point, and made the extremely hopeful request that I could receive a salary advance because I had tax issues and 'various debits' that needed paying off (I asked pointedly that this be kept from the headmaster and to this day I don't know whether it was or not). Remarkably, the salary advance was granted, meaning I received a lower salary in October (when I gambled the whole lot away in a day for the first time) and November. Thinking this could now be a regular thing, I asked again in December, because Christmas was approaching. This time it was declined.

The Bursar, at that point, had told me to ask my bank for a loan instead. In January 2017, I told him that this had been declined, and made my most audacious play yet: asking for a £10,000 loan from the school. Again, it was a 'no' and I was told by the Bursar – an ex-Army officer who took no prisoners – to seek debt counselling from the Citizens Advice Bureau.

My absence from assembly didn't go unnoticed and I was soon summoned to a meeting with the Bursar. In such situations, I was now prone to self-sabotage, because in a sick way I wanted to inflict pain on myself as punishment for my stupidity. So I lied. I denied all knowledge. I claimed that the only feasible explanation was that I'd parked under some low-hanging branches at the tournament that may have caused a little bit of damage. He was slightly taken aback by my response and proceeded to tell me that there were in fact trackers fitted to every bus and that a further investigation would take place to ascertain what had happened. This should have prompted me to own up, but I continued to lie, in the deluded belief that I could still get away with it.

I received plenty of quizzing from colleagues about the bus, which was the talk of the school – an insular environment, just like my last. I got through the morning, before spending the afternoon in my flat, distracting myself with relentless gambling. I was very short on funds after my shocking day on Wednesday, but also had even more motivation to get a big win now because I feared having to pay for the damage to the bus. I tried to be strategic, placing many multiples (a multiple is any bet that includes more than one selection) and backing long shots. I came agonisingly close, but it didn't work. Unsurprisingly, I drank heavily that day, too.

The bus incident wasn't just going to slip away. Had I just reported it straight away, I would have received a slap on the wrist. But I'd lied, and continued to do so. They looked at the tracker, spoke to other teachers and eventually the boys, too. They even looked at CCTV footage. Five days after the incident, on my 30th birthday, all this was laid out to me. Every step of the way, my guilt was obvious. Eventually, in another meeting at the end of term, I admitted that I lied. I'd never felt lower, or more stupid. I wondered why on earth I'd lied. I knew the consequences would be dreadful, but was unable to bring myself to tell the truth.

Throughout the Easter holidays, this hung over me horribly. I told Charlotte that something was up, that there had been an incident with a minibus, but not the extent of the problem. I was actually very keen now to own up about everything, including the gambling, but just had no idea how to.

By the time I returned to school at the start of the summer term – just my third term there – my reputation was in tatters. I'd received a written warning and was banned from driving the minibus temporarily, but was in much more trouble than that. The school's leaders thought me a shambles. They knew nothing of my gambling or mental health issues and were surprised by my behaviour. My mates on the staff made fun of me, unable to understand why I'd lied about something so trivial, but their words stung badly.

Things didn't improve. At the start of May, my dad got in touch. Increasingly, I only really spoke to my parents about Charlotte and how great things were with her, to keep them off the scent. I certainly hadn't told them about the minibus business. My troubles the previous year – and the money they had spent helping me out – meant they would check in with me very often, though.

This time, Dad said he would be nearby for a conference at another school and wanted to see me. I wriggled, saying it wouldn't be possible because of my timetable and the busy cricket season, but he was persistent – adamant, even – that we meet. I arranged some teaching cover and went to meet him in a car park near school, so we could wander into the village for a coffee.

What I didn't realise was that it wasn't just him I was meeting. When I turned the corner into the car park, I saw him stood there with the colleague with whom I'd shared an office at my old school – the same colleague I'd borrowed money from regularly, who had grown increasingly suspicious of my behaviour and had alerted my parents to the dubious loans the year before.

I went white as a sheet and my first instinct was to turn on my heels and flee. But knowing that really there was no escape, I flung my arms around Dad and burst into tears. We decided that a coffee wasn't appropriate and nor was being anywhere near school, so headed into some woods not too far away to walk and talk. My former colleague began explaining why he was there, but I knew already. It was because of the many loans I'd taken from parents at his school. He didn't know the full extent but he knew there were plenty.

There was plenty they could have been here to quiz me on. Over the recent Easter holidays, I'd done a bit to arrest my financial crisis. After my skiing holiday with Charlotte, I'd run some cricket coaching courses through my new club, where I was player/coach. I was paid by them to coach and, somehow, had got them to agree to pay my full fee for the two-year contract in advance. It was a hefty wedge, and very helpful.

My change of cricket clubs had come about in, by now, my usual regrettable and messy fashion. Because I still owed Horspath money, I had said I would continue to play for them for the time being. But I'd been flaky, and not kept up with my repayments. When it came to the first game of pre-season, travel seemed a pain, and my heart just wasn't in it.

A local club heard that I'd moved close by, and made a quiet approach to see if I would like to get involved. I would coach and play but I was in it for all the wrong reasons, with the only draw being the payment. I got a few runs that summer, but I was no use really. I was unreliable, erratic and I put little effort into my game. I would turn up late for matches and miss training for no reason, even though I was the coach. I was overweight, which meant I came to hate bowling – previously always my strong suit – because it was hard work. Perhaps worst of all was the fact that I knew I was still a very good player at this level, and occasionally turned on the style by smashing a hundred or putting in a match-winning performance. The trouble was, I didn't try very often.

So the cricket courses I ran that Easter were a massive help financially, as was an incident driving back from our skiing holiday. We found ourselves stuck at Calais in huge queues caused by issues at immigration. It was Grand National day and, while I'd very little cash left after the holiday, I'd received some payments for the coaching course over the previous couple of days. I put them all on the winner, One For Arthur, which earned me more than £3,000 that helped me make it through the rest of the holidays, both from a living and gambling perspective.

I'd also managed to secure an interest-free loan from the Professional Cricketers' Association (PCA). I received an email from them one day, just a random mailing list update, and it occurred to me that I might be eligible for the sort of help I'd heard they provided to former professional players. I didn't think I fitted the bill as my career had been so short and I was very embarrassed to contact them, but I was desperate, and felt I'd exhausted almost every other avenue. I chanced it, using the end of the tax year as my excuse, explaining that I'd been hit with a huge bill. They said they could help, offering me a £6,000 loan that I would pay back monthly.

But it all went into a bigger and bigger black hole. Before the win that Easter I'd approached more parents from my old school for loans and had crossed another big line – asking parents I didn't even know that well now. After my conversation with my previous headmaster the day I met Charlotte, I'd tried hard to avoid speaking to people connected to the school. But desperation shortened my memory. Less than a term after he issued his warning, I asked half a dozen parents and a couple of them obliged. As an indication of that desperation I asked a parent I thought wouldn't keep my request to himself – but still emailed him anyway.

Back to the woods. Having explained the situation as gently as he could, my old colleague tactfully headed off to give my dad and I some time together alone. The last time showdown talks like this had taken place, seven months earlier, my dad had become aware of some of my debt – but only to financial institutions and people I knew personally. Now he discovered that I'd crossed an ethical boundary in an industry he held so dear. That I was desperate was obvious to him, but he was horrified. I had no choice but to accept I'd made some terrible decisions. I pretty much hadn't stopped crying since first clapping eyes on him that day.

I felt even lower now than I had about the minibus incident a few weeks earlier. It was the closest I came to a total meltdown and revealing everything. But I was just too fearful of the consequences to go through with it. I admitted that I'd approached these people for help, but denied that I'd received money from many of them. I said I knew what I'd done was wrong and that I would never do it again.

Rejoining my old colleague, we agreed on the walk back to the car that he would keep a closer eye on me on my parents' behalf. Given previous conversations, they knew that gambling was involved. But I was adamant that I only used it as an occasional stress reliever, and that while I'd lost some bets on a rare recent binge, the financial situation had improved. They believed any previous debts had been repaid in full. However, this could not have been further from the truth. In fact, any money that had been given to me to repay my historic debts (including the bank loan my dad had taken out) had almost all been gambled away. By now, my debts were probably approaching six figures.

Believing what I said, they both made me promise that I would stop gambling even in the small amounts I was admitting to, and I agreed. It was a surprise to me that I had managed to appear convincing and trustworthy enough to get this response. But I had become a masterful liar.

I wanted nothing more than to be able to keep my word. To be able to stop gambling. For the first time, after all these years as a secret addict, I wanted to stop, and I wanted it to stop. The problem was by now that I couldn't cope with the consequences of revealing everything.

By the end of our walk in the woods I'd convinced my dad that I would step back into line, and arranged a follow-up meeting in a week's time. I'd shown more emotion than usual, and made some strong commitments. I'll never forget saying goodbye to them both that afternoon. I wanted to bare my soul even more, but just couldn't. I wanted to stop gambling, but just couldn't. Minutes after they left, when I was alone, despite everything I felt and had said, I was placing bets again. Each one made me feel so sick, angry, despondent and helpless. It made me hate myself even more. My suicidal thoughts were growing stronger.

At the end of that day, I vowed that tomorrow was the day I would stop gambling. I spoke to Dad that night but only felt worse because I knew I'd lied to him. The following day, the day I was supposed to stop, was more of the same. I kept gambling. I would tell myself that this was my final day as a gambler. But I never could stop.

It hurt so much because I knew I was lying and letting people who cared about me down. I had an amazing family, and all they wanted to do was help. And I was grateful that my former colleague was giving up his time to try to help me and my family, all at a time when I still owed him money. He was that kind of guy, and I was lucky to have him in my life. I did feel, though, like a marked man. I left the meeting knowing full well that my old school was now a no-go zone for financial help. My old colleague was on red alert. Over the months that followed, I became very wary of him, and pushed him away.

So I was now in deep trouble at my old school and my current school. I was making awful decisions that felt totally beyond my control. The minibus damage should have been a wake-up call – it had shown that gambling and my desperation to place a bet and watch a race could cloud even the simplest judgement and set in train a disastrous sequence of events. But I just couldn't stop.

And now another lucrative financial avenue was closed off – parents at my old school, just like the bank and payday loans before them. But I still needed money. By now it wasn't at all unusual for my entire salary to be spent in the 24 hours after it landed – although sometimes I would still win big early in the month, sustaining me. I had to keep Charlotte off the scent too, so having some money was doubly important.

I was on edge and was being closely watched at school but with the headmaster gone and senior staff holding such a low opinion of me, I didn't really care any more. I just wanted to keep my head above water, nothing else.

Since the spring half-term trip to Cape Town, I'd grown close to parents at my new school. Now we were into the cricket season, I was spending more time with them around matches, and growing increasingly confident in their company. Despite telling my dad and old colleague that asking for loans was all behind me, I decided to take the plunge and ask a couple of parents for money. I figured I was less likely to be busted, because my old colleague had no way of policing me at a school he didn't work in. That showed how warped my thinking was: if borrowing from parents at a school I'd left was risky (and unethical), to do so at my current school was another level entirely. If I was found out, I would surely be sacked instantly.

I used the same approach as I had previously – contacting them via email, asking for strict confidence and for it not to be discussed at school. I would tell them about a big tax bill or a broken car. Again, it worked, and I agreed repayment terms with those who lent me cash.

This time there was a difference, though. I was still teaching these people's kids, so I was seeing them regularly. My previous creditors had been at an arm's length. They were out of sight and out of mind. But now I would run into them at a cricket match or in a school corridor, and be dreading conversations about the 'special' relationship we had struck up. I began actively avoiding them, walking in the opposite direction if I spotted them out of the corner of my eye. Having said that, it didn't stop me asking more and more of them for money as the months passed. I was that desperate.

Some of the loans I took from individuals were now very significant, as much as £10,000 a pop. With some of them, I sustained myself day to day. With others, I paid off some of the interest on the most painful payday loans, which was a rare moment of clear-headed good sense. With most of it though, I just gambled. Truly, without the support of Charlotte and my family, I would have been ready to take my own life then. It was all that was stopping me. I hated myself, hated the world, hated my behaviour. I was utterly helpless.

11

August 2017

By the time Charlotte moved in with me in the summer holidays, in August, it was clear that my web of lies was close to being exposed. And mentally and physically, I was hanging on by a thread. My suicidal thoughts continued, so I went to see my GP. I was prescribed antidepressants. I kept this from everyone, including Charlotte.

In a twist I couldn't make up if I tried, the flat we were moving into was opposite a Coral betting shop. I was already among their most valued customers, and there were also two pubs, each 50 yards either side of the flat. I was in both pretty often as well. To top it off, there was a nearby Tesco with a cashpoint outside. Every time I went to the supermarket to get supplies, I would withdraw cash (if my balance would allow me to), and nip into Coral. The implications for an addict are obvious.

Charlotte:

It felt like exactly the right time to move in together. We had been going out for about nine months by the time the big day came and it all felt very natural.

We had wanted to be able to spend more time together, rather than just seeing each other a couple of times a week. I was also saving up for a house, so no longer paying rent was convenient, too.

What wasn't convenient was that I was now driving 80 miles every day to and from my job. I would be out of the house by 6 a.m. and wouldn't return until after 6 p.m. – on a good day. So while we saw much more of each other, especially on the weekend (although he worked Saturdays), it wasn't the constant company that some couples enjoy. His job was ever more demanding time-wise the more settled and senior he became.

We started to get into a routine and the rhythms of living together though. At the weekend, when he was working, I would relax, or do boring but necessary bits around the flat. When he finished work, we would go on trips to all the lovely towns and villages in that lovely part of the world, and enjoy pub food. We were still pretty new so were getting to know each other's friends, too. It was an exciting time.

I'd lived with another partner a few years earlier, so it wasn't the totally new experience for me that it was for Patrick. He adapted pretty well, and he was much the same hard-working, fun man that I'd got to know in the previous few months. Of course, there were a few little things, but nothing out of the ordinary.

A few old habits died hard. There were times on a Saturday where he'd be coaching sport and we would have agreed to have a takeaway that evening. He would go for the customary couple of pints with his colleagues and end up rolling in pissed – coherent but clearly well-oiled – long after dinner time. It wasn't disgraceful behaviour, but it was inconsiderate and frustrating.

Like all his weaknesses, I felt they were explainable and excusable. He was still getting used to living with a partner for the first time, and all the extra considerations that brings. They were the kind of things that would piss me off briefly, but weren't major issues.

I expected a bit better of him and did find it odd when he dropped below those standards – I suppose you could say when he let me down, if you were being harsh – but he would

always make up for it. He knew when he'd drunk too much
and would be very hard on himself, and therefore very good
to me. The bad bits irritated me, but it was nothing more
than you'd expect any other couple to go through, and it was
certainly worth it because his standout features were that he
was generous and loving.

Moving in with Charlotte felt grown up, and I really loved her
so it was wonderfully exciting. It felt so right, and yet I was also
highly apprehensive because I knew that I was getting myself
into something unsustainable. I moved all her stuff myself to
save money, and got some gap-year students from school to
help me out. I took them for a few beers to say thanks.

At the end of August, just before we went back to school, we
went on holiday with my family. It was low-key, and everyone
had a lovely time. It should have been relaxing, but I was racked
with guilt that I was lying to everybody around me in so many
different ways.

I relished the return of school, and the much-needed structure
it provided. I loved coaching rugby, which was one of my main
jobs at this time of year, and now it was term-time I didn't have
as many outgoings, because I could scrounge school meals. I'd
taken on some extra responsibility, so was almost at the same
position I'd been at my previous school. Just like my ability to
lie and appear so convincing about my financial situation, I was
somehow able to maintain a professional front, which meant
my teaching ability was rarely questioned. It seems implausible
that I was able to pull this off, but I could.

A few quid saved on lunch doesn't mean that this autumn
wasn't an extremely damaging time financially, though – as
usual. Although I'd taken a bit of time to settle in a year earlier,
it wasn't because I didn't get on with my colleagues. They were
great, and I fitted in straight away. A year on, I'd forged some
strong friendships and, also as usual, I was considered the life

and soul of the party. My troubles had never been spotted by my peers, even if some senior staff knew on a confidential basis that I'd stepped out of line.

But I began to make mistakes. I had a great mate who was single, loved a drink and also enjoyed betting. For a while, we had all three in common. Even after I met Charlotte, we would drink and bet together. He would bet small amounts very often, and I led him to believe that I did the same thing – if anything, less often. A few times I asked him (and other colleagues) if I could borrow some money, but I could tell it bugged him. I was desperate and apologetic, and as a friend he was willing to help, but it did me no favours.

I hit a new low in September when, after being bombarded with online adverts, I became aware of a company called Amigo Loans. I'd exhausted most of my payday loan options some years earlier, and had been juggling the repayments ever since. Amigo (what an ironic name that is!) had very high interest rates, and required a guarantor – who had to be a homeowner – to secure a loan.

I decided that I needed a loan, for £10,000, but knew there was no way I could ask my parents to guarantee it, and Charlotte wasn't a homeowner (not that I could have realistically asked her anyway). Nor were many of my close mates and, anyway, I knew asking them would cause alarm. So I turned to a colleague I got on very well with (a close friend, but not someone I had gambled with before). He was big-hearted, the sort who wanted to help. I assured him that £300 repayments each month were manageable and, with a warning of how serious all this was and the consequences it would have if it went sour, he agreed. I sent him the online paperwork, which he filled out. By the end of the day, I had £10,000 in my account. The fact that I was due to pay back £20,000 seemed irrelevant: I had funds.

I gambled the entire loan in the space of a week.

In one fell swoop, I'd deepened my troubles massively. This would have taken my debt past £125,000. I didn't know what to do. Of course, I didn't tell the colleague or anyone else. Making excuses wasn't easy, and I ran away from communicating with my creditors. I started to ignore letters, particularly anything that said 'Private and Confidential'. I would just rip it up and bin it before reading, because I knew I wouldn't like what I saw. I began to receive emails and texts from companies I'd never heard of, because my loans and debts were being handed to debt collection agencies. My phone would ring with numbers I didn't recognise; as a hater of phone calls already, I was definitely not picking up.

And it's little surprise that they were contacting me. I owed them huge amounts of money. One of the payday loans had risen to 1,497 per cent APR (annual percentage rate). For context, most credit cards sit at about 20 per cent.

The start of each month was doubly uncomfortable, because the individuals I owed – including colleagues and parents – knew that I'd been paid and should, therefore, be in a position to reimburse them. But I was nowhere near that.

Charlotte:

The problems I'd sensed in Patrick's behaviour in the first few months of our relationship did become a little more apparent in the second half of 2017, but they still weren't outrageous or obvious.

There was a time when we were out for a pub lunch and he became very concerned that a colleague from his old school – with whom he was close – was trying to call him. I thought it was odd, especially when he admitted that he owed him a little bit of cash from the last time they had met up. I told him to go outside and take the call, which he did. He'd been so anxious and concerned, but returned calm and saying how kind and supportive the colleague had been.

There were two moments that did stop me in my tracks. One Saturday morning while he was at work, towards the end of the year, I came across something that worried me greatly. I was just knocking about the flat, playing around on an iPad. I thought it was mine, so reflexively went to check my emails. But it was his iPad and his emails. The way he treated his phone, he certainly wouldn't have wanted me to have access to his emails, although he was a little more relaxed around his iPad. I would never have had the opportunity to just be flicking around on his phone.

Without nosing about at all, I found a series of emails – once I saw one, I had to look at the next, and the next, and the next – all about money. Money that Patrick owed people. I didn't know who these people were but there were informal-looking repayment agreements and emails from Patrick about big tax bills he had to pay. One conversation was very clearly recent, but the others were a little older.

Patrick was at school, so I stewed alone at home, wondering what the hell was going on. I messaged him, telling him that I'd accidentally stumbled across some very concerning emails.

When he returned, he was annoyed at me for looking at his iPad. He huffed and puffed a little, but managed to explain it all away. He looked me in the eye and said that his dad knew all about these arrangements, and everything was under control. He said that if I was concerned, I should call his dad straight away for proof that everything was fine. He opened up about some debt issues he'd had in the past, but assured me that everything was being sorted now.

I was highly sceptical, but he was so convincing and spoke with such conviction that I felt I could hardly argue. It felt like he'd used the opportunity to be honest about something that was difficult for him. I almost felt guilty for finding them and stupid for questioning it.

The other moment came when I was doing our washing and came across a betting slip in his pocket. I looked at the amount, £60, and I was quite taken aback. It was on a footballer (Patrick still remembers it as Leroy Sane of Manchester City to score first in a cup game, at odds of 8/1).

I immediately burst into tears and called a friend, even though I wasn't sure what I was upset about. I just knew nothing about gambling, so was full of questions that she couldn't answer. I was more upset by the value than the act of gambling itself. To us, the way we lived our lives, that was a lot of money – especially at odds like that.

All my male friends at uni had gambled, mainly on football, and it seemed pretty regular, although I have no idea how much they were putting on. It didn't feel like they would have been throwing £60 at it.

When he got home, he went for a shower, and when he came out, I confronted him about it. I asked if he ever gambled. He said he did occasionally. I asked how much and how often. He said perhaps £20 each month. So, I asked, why have I just found this?, and placed the slip in front of him, on our bed. He said it was a one-off, but accepted that sometimes he would gamble as much as £100 a month. That felt like quite a lot, but he explained it confidently, and told me how careful he was with what he bet on.

I was left bemused enough by the whole situation that I had told my friend and others, in confidence, about it. I now knew he had a relationship with gambling, but felt comfortable enough to leave it alone. In the weeks that followed, I watched him closely, and saw nothing to worry me enough to take further action.

The longer we lived together and the more I fell in love with Charlotte, the more explicit my lies to her became. And I was less likely to open up to her than ever because losing her would be impossible. We had only been together a year but it felt so much longer. Seeing the disappointment in her eyes when she confronted me about these issues hurt deeply, but also sharpened my resolve to tighten my guard.

There was another similar incident with a colleague around the same time. This colleague, who was a very good friend, had asked to borrow something work-related (if memory serves it was a referee's whistle!) and, without thinking, I told him it was in my top drawer and he was welcome to pop in and take it. He opened the drawer and sitting right at the top was a betting slip from Megabet – a less well-known bookmaker he'd probably never even heard of. Because there wasn't a branch locally (I'd popped in while in a nearby town), I hadn't had time to pick up some pretty significant winnings: I'd received a tip from a connection in the racing world to back a horse called Khun John at 9/1. I'd stuck £250 on, and the horse won. I was set to take home more than two grand.

He was understandably taken aback by the size of my bet and brought it up with me. I told him that he'd misread the slip and that there was a decimal point he'd not seen – I'd only stuck £2.50 on and was due to win £20. I doubt he believed me, but he was the most laid-back person going and never mentioned it again.

As soon as I had time, I drove to the nearest Megabet and collected my winnings. I spent them pretty promptly. When I won cash, I tended to put it in an envelope in my locker at school to try to create some discipline. Generally, it didn't work. I didn't normally have cash, though; I did a lot of my gambling at the Coral outside my flat, and they allowed you to place your winnings in the shop straight into your online account.

*　*　*

I love Christmas, but that year, 2017, it was miserable. I was so pent-up, unable to open up on anything as I felt I'd so much to lose. My parents had some idea of my problems and were desperate to help, but I felt that knowing the full extent would break them.

That Christmas, my brother was in Australia watching the Ashes with friends, which left me bereft and miserable. He was an outlet for me. Not because I would share my problems with him; quite the opposite, actually. The things we did together – drinking beer, chewing the fat and watching sport – were the perfect escape. I was envious of him in Australia, because he was having so much fun, while I wallowed in self-pity at home.

I just about kept a brave enough face on things that family alarm bells didn't ring any more than usual. I simply said I missed my brother. As always, I found an excuse. My relationship with my parents was strained, but I just pushed them away. My mum was clearly struggling with it all, while my relationship with my dad became tricky as he shouldered the 'official' side of keeping an eye on me. He was doing all the right things, but it felt like our relationship had been formalised, as if he was my boss or headmaster (as he'd once been). It felt like my situation was all we ever discussed but that was probably because I closed down every attempt at a conversation about it.

Over the holiday I went to London to meet some friends at Winter Wonderland in Hyde Park. I woke up with no memory of the night whatsoever, but a mate told me that we had had all been enjoying ourselves and catching up over a couple of beers, when I just disappeared – for hours. As can happen at a bar, I ran into another mate and drank aggressively with him, before going AWOL. I finally re-emerged and was, in his words, 'the drunkest man alive'. I was unable to communicate with everyone else, who were getting festively merry but little more. Unsurprisingly, mates were exchanging confused and concerned glances about me. I had no idea where the time had gone.

I also went on a skiing holiday with Charlotte and her dad's family. The only reason I could go was because they paid for our trip, which was incredibly generous. I was, by now, way beyond the stage of being able to book a holiday after a nice win (as I had been able to on our last skiing holiday at Easter); I just had too many outgoings with all my repayments.

On this trip, Charlotte's step-brother, who I hadn't spent long period of times with before, happened to spot me on a betting app on my phone, but fortunately didn't see any incriminating details. We shared a knowing look and he asked what I bet on. I said I had an occasional punt on football with an accumulator and he said he did too. The conversation never went further, and he just assumed I was another 30-year-old bloke who liked a bet every now and then. It's remarkable, really, that this very brief exchange was the closest I ever came to being rumbled gambling on my phone.

On the surface, it was a lovely trip to a beautiful place, doing one of my favourite activities, and a great opportunity to get to know Charlotte's loved ones better. But it was emotional torture. There was no escape from company, no time alone to digest the increasing number of messages I was getting, asking why I was defaulting on repayments to all these people I should never have borrowed from in the first place. I was overwhelmed, and absolutely dreading my return to school, when I would have to face the music. I made a huge effort to ensure that Charlotte's family thought nothing was wrong, but behind the facade, I was falling apart. It was exhausting.

Charlotte:

Christmas time meant we had been together for a year, and we were very settled together, as exhibited by the fact that I did the Christmas shopping on behalf of the two of us. I thought I'd done a pretty good job, but I told Patrick how much it had cost and his face fell. He was pretty taken aback and pissed off that I'd spent what I considered a very normal amount, but his initial disappointment didn't last long and within a day or so he'd transferred the money he owed me.

We had a lovely break. I spent some time with his family in Sussex, which was great, just as it had been on our summer holiday with them. And we went on a skiing trip with my family, which was brilliant. It was a thrill for me to see him settle into my family and bond with my step-brothers.

Around this time, a guy I knew well – and therefore Patrick was getting to know too – confided in me that he'd accrued considerable debt because of his use of his credit card. Patrick had told me that he'd had some problems with debt because of his lifestyle when living in London years before but that he'd got back on track with a bit of help from his parents and a loan. I shared this info with this guy as an example that it wasn't all bad and there was a way out.

There's one other incident from this time that sticks in my mind. I was cleaning out the bathroom in our flat when I came across two packs of tablets tucked away. The first were clearly antidepressants. And the second was to reduce a buildup of stomach acid.

I questioned Patrick on both. I wasn't wildly surprised about the antidepressants. I knew he'd struggled with his mental health, and countering that with medication wasn't uncommon among people our age. He explained that the antidepressants had caused stomach issues.

I'd always had problems with my stomach because my body had always produced a lot of acid. I suffered from heartburn, too. That's not surprising given I was overweight, and drinking and smoking too much. Increasingly often, when I drank (even in moderation), I would be very sick. But things got worse when I was stressed and I'd now developed a stomach ulcer and was on strong medication for it.

It felt to me like Charlotte was sensing that I told lies and kept things from her. That was a major concern, but I had many other worries too. I no longer had parents left at school who I could go to and ask for money. All those I felt close enough to had said a confused 'no', or a reluctant 'yes'. As the emails I was receiving attested, I was really struggling to pay anything back to those in the latter camp. Even the creditors I was most keen to pay back, like the PCA, had to be ignored.

In my spare time, I flicked through my contacts list on my phone, and the hundreds of people I was friends with on Facebook. I would size each up, with two considerations: 1) whether they were in a position to lend to me; and 2) whether my request for cash would get back to my friends and family. Ultimately, though, I wasn't too picky, and sent hundreds of messages, without much success. When people said 'no', I wouldn't take it personally. I would just move on to the next person, until someone said 'yes'.

Inevitably, this only widened the cracks. The people I was approaching found it weird that I was asking for money, and my due diligence wasn't tight enough. These were people I hadn't seen for years, and now had only tenuous links with. I remember learning that a bloke I'd played cricket with for one season now had a decent property business, so asked him for money. He then understandably shared our exchange with a mutual friend, putting them on red alert about my behaviour.

People were beginning to spot things and ask tricky questions of me but, honestly, as 2018 rolled round, I was almost laughing that I was still standing on my own two feet. Not because I found it funny, but because if I didn't laugh, I'd cry. It seemed scarcely believable that I'd got away with it so far. In this whole time, I'd never once been in a situation where I was out for dinner with Charlotte and my card had bounced. Given I was by now surgically attached to it, I'd never been told off – not once – for being on my phone while I taught kids.

*   *   *

In 2017, my gambling had truly run wild. This was the year that I hit 76 different accounts (often having multiple accounts with the same gambling company) and, in one account alone, placed 27,988 bets. I'd built up all these accounts up over the years, and they were in many different names, mainly of people I knew.

I would put in the bare minimum information required, and came to know which companies asked for photo ID. The people whose names I used would, of course, have no idea I was doing this, because I would use my own email addresses (I had at least half a dozen, specifically for this purpose) and make sure there was no way of them receiving marketing communications or anything similar. I had multiple accounts with the same bookmaker so I could back the same races and matches over and over again.

I would flit through the accounts, using them at different times. For some, I'd forgotten the password or even the email address associated with it years before, so they just lay dormant. I don't think I ever actually closed one.

I had phases where I used certain accounts relentlessly because I believed I was on a lucky streak and, like the cricketer who won't move seat while his teammates bat in a nervy run chase, change could bring about a downturn in fortunes. Only when I emptied that account would I move on to the next.

As mentioned before, I also had accounts with VIP status, and would leverage that position for bonuses and freebies, but now I became far more sinister. I became really nasty with them, threatening that I would harm myself if I didn't get what I wanted, or claim that I was about to lose my job. It was pure emotional blackmail. There was one operator with whom I was particularly aggressive, because I knew I would get what I wanted. They almost all said yes in the end. And why not? I would end up giving them all of my money anyway.

Very occasionally I would receive some form of concerned communication from an operator, because I'd made worrying comments that triggered whatever duty of care they had in place. They would reference account management tools or self-exclusion options, or signpost some support. But ultimately it was left to me to action these, which I was never going to do.

I would gamble on every single horse race at every meet throughout the day, and just about every football league match (bear in mind there are 92 clubs). Saturdays, as you can imagine, were carnage – I would put quite literally thousands of bets on, either placed in preparation overnight or just on my phone on the day. Thursday afternoons, my half-day from school, were similar.

I would get angry when I had a winning bet that had not landed in my account by the time I wanted to place my next one. The gap between a bet winning and the winnings being paid was only ever a few minutes, yet it was still much too long for me.

Managing these accounts was at times like having yet another full-time job. I had no concept of what was going in and out of them. You can deposit in a matter of seconds, but it takes days to withdraw cash. On the few occasions that I did try to withdraw money this would normally never materialise because any withdrawal would be pending for several days – in which time I could not resist cancelling the withdrawal to gamble it. All this was utterly knackering – and simply brutal.

When my money ran dry and my accounts were empty, I would experience a brief moment of relief. I could do nothing more. But that wouldn't last long – I would go hunting for money once more.

All this gambling was in search of the salvation that was the 'big win'. By now, I knew it would need more than just one extraordinary bet to get me out of trouble, but I honestly thought it would happen. I came close to huge wins on massive multiples that left me feeling like the unluckiest man alive. They also just kept me coming back for more.

It had been an astonishing year. But really, 2017 was just the calm before the storm.

12

January 2018

I'd always dreaded returning to school after the holidays. After Christmas was always the worst. January is a tough month financially and emotionally for most people, with short days and bitter weather.

I was unable – not just financially but also mentally – to keep up with the repayments for the many loans I now had. My 'friends' at Amigo Loans were particularly punishing with their demands for repayments, and their interest rates. There were certain loans that I was desperate to repay purely on a human level, such as to the PCA and many parents at school, but on a practical level, I just could not keep up.

My monthly salary wouldn't even cover a quarter of the repayments I owed, let alone basic living expenses and the exorbitantly costly gambling addiction I was living with. I'd so many people contacting me about defaulted payments and I'd approached so many new people about borrowing from them over the holidays.

My approach to funding my addiction – which almost exclusively amounted to borrowing – was totally scattergun. I was struggling to know who to repay first, or indeed who to ask for money next. I was desperately approaching people who I'd lost touch with (people I went to school with, or big hitters from the city that I hadn't seen for years), but that led to more questions than answers. Naturally they almost all said 'no', but they also contacted mutual friends asking two questions – what the hell is going on; and, has he asked to borrow from you? I hadn't asked closer friends because I thought that was the likeliest way my web of lies would be exposed. The questions continued.

I returned to school feeling like I was about to face the music from parents of kids I taught who I'd not paid back. I feared that someone would have told the school, or that I would be confronted in a corridor about what had gone on. I scheduled another cricket coaching course in April, which would bring in more cash. This time, I was less patient, and insisted that the kids signing up had to be paid for in advance. It worked a treat, and I'd more than 100 kids locked in some three months before the event. It just about kept me going.

On a Wednesday in the second week of term, I'd another issue while on a school bus on the way to a sports fixture. The night before, I'd received a message from my tipster, who suggested that I might want to back a horse called Dichato, ridden by one of my favourite jockeys, Richard Kingscote, at lunchtime the following day at Lingfield Park. The odds were 13/8. I was unable to say no.

The trouble was that, as so often, I'd no funds to place the bet. As was customary now, I responded to the tip by contacting two parents at the school, both of whom I'd borrowed from before. In my email that evening, asking for money, I would by now always request an exact figure, based on gut feel, informed by whether I'd borrowed from them before and what I thought they could afford to realistically lend. I would cite debt consolidation, saying I was very nearly in the clear financially. I promised big, fast repayments to show my confidence. Each of these emails was a direct risk to my job. The school would be mortified if they had known.

I was asking for bigger amounts these days as I was so tired of the stress that came with asking people for money. I just wanted large amounts so fewer conversations were involved, even though those conversations that did take place were so painful because of the high stakes involved.

Anyway, I asked one parent for a large amount – a few thousand – and the other for double that. The first emailed back that night, agreeing to the deal. The money was transferred promptly. The other, an intimidating and influential guy, didn't email me back that evening. He waited until the morning, and we spoke on the phone, which I couldn't bear. On this occasion the pain of the call was worth it. The conversation, at break time, was desperately difficult, not least when he made a throwaway comment about me needing the money to pay 'gambling debts'. I laughed nervously, and said of course it wasn't – it was debt consolidation. He let it lie, but his message was pretty simple and forceful: do not screw this up. I was in total disbelief that I had managed to pull off this request and he transferred the money soon after.

Confident, I piled £8,000 on Dichato across multiple gambling accounts, then another £2,000 on multiples including the same horse, before heading to a sports fixture at another school. It was unusual that I was spreading my bets around all these different accounts because increasingly I just laid big bets on the nose, which showed how reckless and greedy I now was. I put some of these bets on each way – meaning I would win something if it came second or third – to feel on the safe side.

This time, we were on a coach, not a minibus. The teachers sat near the front, with the boys chattering away behind us. I made sure I had two seats to myself so I could enjoy the race on my phone with my headphones in when really I should have been chatting to my colleagues or the kids, or doing some work. The school had policies for staff phone use, and by now I defied them every single day.

The race was a disaster. Dichato came fourth – meaning I won nothing, despite hedging my bets. It was made worse when I realised that a child who was sitting behind me had spent the race alternating between peering through the gap between the seats and watching in the window's reflection. As I was coming to terms with my latest catastrophic loss, he asked innocently if my horses had won.

Just like on the minibus 10 months earlier, I didn't see the funny side, and he seemed surprised, because that was just not the kind of teacher I was. I spent the remainder of the journey with my jacket over my head, pretending to sleep. In reality, I was in tears.

Looking back, it's this incident that makes me most sad – more than any in my gambling journey, in fact. There were other moments in which I had behaved worse and lost more but none that had such an impact as this. It was a trigger for my descent into total free fall. You might think I'd been in that state for some time, but I went to another level now. I hit the self-destruct button. This highlights the extent of my addiction: just when I had reached a low ebb and felt I could not go on, I would find a way to debase myself further. The shame associated with each unforgiveable act fed the next act of debasement.

On a basic level, I was another £10,000 deeper into debt, with more than half of it owed to a man who had been quite clear that he suspected the root of my problem and that he wasn't going to tolerate any bullshit from me. I now had to get hold of some money – fast – and my approach to borrowing became even more wild and wayward. My focus was repaying him, ignoring other debts, because this really felt like the one that would bring everything crashing down.

The value of money itself was gone, which was why I was able to ask for such obscene amounts from people I barely knew. Money didn't have any meaning – apart from to feed my greedy addiction. And the outcome of my bets only actually mattered now because they either allowed me to bet more, or not.

I'd become ever more socially reclusive and unreliable. I no longer arranged to meet up with many of my mates and was dreadful at committing to activities, mainly because I never knew until a few minutes before if I could afford to attend. But there was an element of social anxiety too, a fear that I would be confronted in public about the ridiculous requests for money I was making, or even asked directly about gambling.

And yet my borrowing became ever riskier. I started to approach friends' parents, which was clearly exceptionally stupid, while a couple of my other requests made their way back to my brother in Oxford. I could just about wriggle out of it, and made sure I told the person I'd asked that no, I didn't need the money, I'd sorted the issue out.

There were now people in my life – including my brother and some close friends – worrying about me, and asking if I was OK. Of course, I said I was fine when I was anything but. I felt my family and friends were closer to rumbling me, and so was the gambling industry. I was bombarding them with requests for free bets, and guilt-tripping them as I had done for some time. I even told them I was considering taking my life because of gambling, which was true, but I wasn't telling them this in order to get help, I was telling them because I wanted freebies.

In response, I started to receive more communication from some – not all – bookmakers, signposting how I could self-exclude from their app and website, and how I could get help for gambling addiction. If they had been paying attention, they would have known for some time that I was a gambling addict but they continued to allow me to bet. Now I was a problem they could no longer ignore. In a couple of cases, my account was shut down, or limited. If a bookmaker is telling you to stop, it might be time to listen.

I didn't, of course. I wasn't interested and refused to engage. Most of their communication came via email, but they did try to call. I wouldn't pick up the phone to my parents at this stage, let alone a bookie.

My appetite for alcohol continued to grow, but it became less social. I would drink on the sly, telling no one that I was off to the pub. I never drank on the job, but I would have a Stella in my hand promptly when my school day finished. Having been a sportsman all my life, I was doing the square root of nothing for my physical health. I ate junk, and did no exercise. My sleep was worse than ever. I would stay up gambling, or scrambling around, looking for loans. My mind just wouldn't stop whirring.

In February half-term I went on a colleague's stag do to Newcastle. I couldn't afford it, so spent the days before doing a huge recruitment drive for my coaching course at half-term, with some success. My behaviour was wild, and I was considered the perfect stag do guest, guzzling pints and leading the charge, even though I was slipping off for plenty of alone-time away from the group. The group was full of sporty lads who liked a punt, and there was a lot of sport on that weekend, including the Six Nations, so gambling was a hot topic. I organised big group bets, which helped cover the fact that I'd a problem – it seemed like I was doing it for the greater good. All my behaviour was an act and it caught up with me on a horrendous drive home. I cried all the way.

It was hard to hide my mental state during half-term from Charlotte, but I made it through. I wanted to show as few cracks as possible. In term time, I felt bad for her about the time she spent commuting and the lengths of her workdays. But if I'm honest, it bought me time with myself. When I didn't go to the pub, I would get home from school before her and let my emotion out. I would lie on the bed or in the bath and just cry, before pulling myself together for her return. I was tired all the time, and drank an obscene amount of coffee.

My mental health was worse than ever. I considered quitting my job and walking away – who knows where. There were times when I was driving when I wondered whether it was possible for me to just veer sharply off the road to see what would happen. If I died, so be it. I remember catching a train and standing on the edge of the platform, weighing up whether that would be a plausible way to go, too.

The gap between each suicidal thought became ever shorter. I had to remember that I'd an extraordinary family, who let me know often how much they cared about me – despite me pushing them away. It was them, and Charlotte, who kept me from taking my life. I would have done it in a heartbeat otherwise, because I felt worthless in every way. I saw no way to stop gambling and no way out of my financial issues. My faith that the big win was round the corner had diminished.

Addiction to gambling made me feel totally alone. I knew people who were increasingly open about their depression and anxiety, but I didn't know anyone else who had suffered what I was going through. Why was no one else in this situation? Why only me? I felt like I should be able to just stop gambling. I wanted to, and had tried, but I couldn't. Even now, it's actually hard to explain how gripped I was.

I'd had moments when I considered telling people. I did visit my GP again. I'd been on medicine for my mental health since the previous spring, but needed more now. In a cry for help, I told the doctor that I was suicidal, that it was my gambling that drove these feelings, and that I had a lot of debt. I didn't feel like there was a great deal of understanding (or empathy) about what I was describing. They moved fast to deal with the depression and anxiety I described, but pretty much ignored that I'd mentioned gambling. That only strengthened my sense that there wasn't much that could be done about all this. I was fucked until I died.

I was, to be fair, prescribed stronger antidepressants and sleeping pills, both of which helped my state of mind a little bit. Still, each day was a battle and it felt like success just to make it through. Because I slept so badly, every day just yawned into the next with no break whatsoever. But now, rather than waking up wondering if today was the day that I would place the bet that would save me, I woke up wondering if this was the day that would see my world come crashing down, and everything exposed.

Through all this, there was one remarkable development: I got a promotion. I applied for a job as Head of Year and somehow got it. I almost didn't go for it because I felt guilty and a complete fraud, but was encouraged to. My experience of the role in a larger school won me the role. It seemed completely farcical to me, given my disciplinary record and the meltdown I was experiencing (although they didn't know about that bit). I was clearly still able to turn it on when I needed to, and it helped convince others that I was OK. The one thing that could never be questioned, and made me stand out from my colleagues, was my rapport with the kids. This, along with my natural disposition, and the fact that I continued to do what was required of me did not go unnoticed.

I told Charlotte, but couldn't bring myself to celebrate. I was convinced that by the time I was due to take up the role a couple of months later, I would be sacked, in prison or perhaps even dead.

When my next pay packet (of around £2,000) landed, I did a little calculation. I worked out that to meet all the repayment instalments I owed for March 2018 – just that one month – to individuals, payday loan companies, banks and credit cards I would have need £43,964.

I did some work patching up the situation, which I considered quite clever, contacting people I owed informing them that I needed emergency dental care at short notice – this was rubbish, of course – and so I was unable to make my repayment this month. Many were very understanding and it got them off my back.

Not all were, though, and I was still spraying out so many requests for money and my behaviour was so risky that the emails I received in response became ever more painful. Why are you approaching me for money? Why have you not paid me back? Are you lying to me? Each one was like being punched. Walking round school at the beginning and end of the day, when parents were around, was hellish, because around every corner there was someone I was running away from.

I did make some repayments, those that I felt I simply couldn't avoid. They included Amigo Loans, partly because of the astronomical interest rates, and partly because failing to keep up would see them alert the guarantor. I paid anyone who was chasing me up, anyone I feared, and the few with whom I had written contracts. Those repayments left me with nothing to live on, or gamble. So the cycle of borrowing continued.

And my friends' parents I contacted? They just informed me that they would help in any way possible, but not financially, and then flagged the issue with their kids – my friends – who then raised it with me. At the same time, my friends started to have quiet conversations with my family.

There was nowhere left for me to go. Except it was now March, and that meant one thing: Cheltenham.

13

March 2018

Standing on platform 5 at Slough station, I was certain of two things – that I'd placed my last bet, and that I was about to take my last breath. I would only end up following through with one of them.

I was a mess. Onlookers appeared confused by the sight of a 6ft 2in, thick-set, flame-haired man smartly dressed but in floods of tears and unable to stand still. No one came over, though. Perhaps they assumed I had just said a particularly tricky goodbye. In reality, I was preparing to say goodbye to everything.

I was gripped by the thought that I hadn't told anyone about the trouble I was in. Those close to me deserved some sort of explanation. At the very least there would be people wondering where I'd gone. But I was also ready to go – and there was too much to explain and far too little time to do so.

As a peace-keeping compromise with myself, I fired off two WhatsApp messages. I couldn't call the recipients, because I didn't want them to hear the state I was in, or for that to be their final memory of me.

The first was to Charlotte. I simply wrote: 'I do not want to be here anymore. I'm sorry. X.'

The other was to my brother. We were very close, but he had no sense of the extent to which I was suffering, because I had said nothing. A couple of people had raised vague concerns about me to him, but our relationship was happy and based on fun. I also knew he would have his phone in his hand, because he was always glued to the thing. So as well as being my brother, he was perhaps the most likely person in my whole phonebook to read it promptly.

I didn't tell him exactly where I was, but told him what I was thinking about doing. I said my situation was dire, and asked him to say goodbye to everyone and tell them that I loved them. As I predicted he would, my brother read the message almost immediately, whereas Charlotte – busy in her work as a teacher – didn't. I saw the two blue ticks next to the WhatsApp message but he didn't reply and, in my scrambled mind, thought that he must have agreed with what I'd typed. I thought he wanted me to jump in front of the train. In fact, he'd just read the hardest few words he had – and hopefully will – ever read in his life.

Three minutes passed, and an announcement went out informing people on the platform to stand back because the oncoming train wouldn't be stopping. I was bracing myself to jump when my phone started to go mad in my pocket. My brother was trying to call me, but my mind was made up: I wasn't going to answer.

Still holding my phone, a reply to my WhatsApp popped up. He said that he had no idea what was going on, but whatever I'd done, this was not the solution. He said that if I went ahead and did this, he and the rest of my family wouldn't be able to cope. He said that I could talk to him about anything.

He didn't know I was at the station, or how close I really was to taking my own life. Perhaps he would have reacted differently and panicked even more if he knew. But I truly believe his words were the only things I could have read that stopped me in my tracks the way they did. His message gave me perspective, and reminded me that this wasn't all about me. Until now, I hadn't considered the devastation I would leave behind. I'd just thought everything would be simpler without me.

It reminded me of my two brushes with death I'd experienced in recent years. First, in the taxi in Cape Town. The driver, who lay dead next to me that night, had never been able to say goodbye to his loved ones. I was lucky to walk away from that tragedy with a second chance at life.

The second was the death of the headmaster – my boss, friend and mentor. The pain experienced by those even closer to him, his incredible family, was even more devastating. How could I put my loved ones through that, without an explanation? The headmaster's motto, which he said every day, was 'everything's going to be all right'. Now was the moment to channel that.

So, still in floods of tears, I stepped back, took a deep breath and, moments later, watched the train go past on its way to London. I'd made so many bad decisions, but this was the best one I would ever make. I thought about all the mammoth obstacles that I'd been running away from, and now had to face. But, for the first time in maybe a decade, I felt a sense of relief. I felt good. I'd finally told someone that I had issues I couldn't deal with alone. I'd owned up. Perhaps now I could get the help that I needed so badly, but had resisted for so long.

I slowly walked back to my car (I'd not even received a parking ticket!). Before opening the door, I was violently sick. It was a combination of all those pills, the alcohol from the night before, and the emotional turmoil I'd put myself through.

As I had on the way there, I took a round-about route home. I spent almost two hours gathering my thoughts and, by the time I got home, my brother had got hold of Charlotte, who had had the shock of her life and had left work as soon as she read my message, and my parents. It was decided that Charlotte would look after me while my brother spoke to my parents, because I couldn't have too many people around me so soon after such trauma.

Before Charlotte arrived home, I took the first steps to picking up the pieces of my life. I tidied away the remaining pills – I'd taken quite a lot of the 97 – and the smashed piggy bank. I had a shower and sat on the sofa, still shaking, waiting for her.

I was hollowed out when she returned. She ran over, we embraced and I apologised. I wasn't ready to see my parents, so asked her to delay their arrival by 24 hours, which I spent most of sat in a dark room, with the TV on but not being watched. I'd taken so many sleeping pills earlier that I couldn't stay awake. In hindsight, I probably should have gone to hospital, but I could not face leaving home.

Charlotte waited – both on me and for me. There was no pressure. All I wanted was an assurance that she wasn't walking away immediately, and she gave me that. She was extraordinary. With the help of all those pills, I slept deeply that night, in a way that I'd not for a long time.

I was broken. I replayed moments from that month and the last few years in my head. Thinking about it for the first time, the magnitude of it all struck me. I felt deep fear and shame. My parents arrived the following morning, and my hug with Mum felt like it lasted a lifetime. The four of us sat around a table and I bared my soul to three of the most important people in my life over the course of more than five hours. I told them everything – the lies, the debts, the fact I would inevitably lose my job and the house that came with it, even the looming possibility of time in prison. Even now, it took me some time to open up about the extent of my financial issues. I said it was so bad that I couldn't tell them, but they kept pushing. I didn't know an exact figure, but I knew a ballpark. Crying and shaking, I finally told them. We looked at it all in more detail, and came across loans and credit cards that I'd totally forgotten about. There were that many.

I'd lied so many times on the phone, trying to prise money from people I barely knew. But this was by far the hardest conversation I'd ever had, the toughest thing I'd ever had to do. I never wanted to have this conversation because when I'd played the scenario out in my head, the response was anger, shame and pain. There was a stigma attached to gambling, and certainly to what I'd done as a result of my gambling. I would be screamed at and disowned. Those thoughts never added up to the truth, though, because all three people I was speaking to were calm, compassionate and kind people who loved me. To react like that is not in their nature. We all cried, a lot, as the emotion I'd been locking up flowed out.

Of course, they weren't pleased, or proud of how I'd behaved. And, of course, they recognised that I was significantly damaged and that huge challenges lay ahead for me. But there was clear relief: I'd reached out before it was too late. I was still there, in front of them. I was suffering from an illness, but help was available. They agreed to support me in any way possible, on one condition: that I did everything I could to stop gambling and that I accepted all the help offered.

I was at the very start of a new journey. Even though I'd come clean, I had no idea how I could stop gambling, or what was next. Recovering from addiction was complicated enough, but managing all the trouble I'd caused in the last few years added layer after layer of difficulty.

I did have to make some significant immediate changes. Within a few hours of stepping back from the platform, I'd deleted all gambling apps from my phone. Over the weekend, I contacted the gambling accounts that remained active, and requested to be excluded by the bookmakers, which was promptly done and they provided some practical barriers to stop me getting back in, such as blocking software on all devices (I couldn't access their websites or apps). It helped that I was surrounded – and watched like a hawk – by Charlotte, Mum and Dad all weekend. I couldn't have used my phone for any nefarious means even if I'd wanted to. At night, my phone was kept in another room, and I actually slept. I took every step to stay away from it.

That Saturday afternoon, I spoke on the phone to Mandy Saligari, with whom Mum had already been in contact. Mandy ran a treatment centre in London and had had her own battle with addiction many years earlier. Instantly, I felt she was speaking a language I understood.

She told me that treatment wouldn't work if I was being forced into it by others. The programme was abstinence-based and I had to embrace stopping gambling immediately. Only I could make myself stop, and I had to want it. And I did want nothing more than to never see another bookmakers' shop or betting slip in my life. I knew this would take huge stocks of resolve, and wouldn't simply happen by itself. But that basic determination was there; I'd been given another chance and couldn't mess it up.

I was obsessively worrying, especially about the cost of all this. My parents had already spent so much money on me and I'd frittered it away. They assured me that a way would be found, but the cost was a thought that never left me, and acted as further motivation to quit.

By the time I was admitted to Mandy's clinic on Monday, our lives had already undergone significant changes. On Sunday, knowing what was coming, we started moving out of the house owned by the school, so Charlotte and I moved temporarily to Oxford, where my heavily pregnant older sister, her husband and young daughter still lived on-site at the school I'd worked at two years earlier. It was the Easter holidays, so the two of us, and my parents, moved into dormitories in the boarding house attached to their place. My brother was also still living nearby.

On Monday, Mum accompanied me to the clinic, and as we filled out the forms, both of us were in floods of tears – I felt like an 11-year-old starting a new school. She picked me up at the end of the day, because the programme was non-residential. I was on an Intensive Outpatient Programme, meaning I was getting support in a protected environment but wasn't shut away and still had to maintain a 'normal' life. It gave me daily contact with my family, which I needed.

After day one, I was trusted to commute back and forth on the Oxford Tube bus service. Mum, Dad or Charlotte would drop me at the bus, buy me a ticket, then give me £10 to get myself lunch.

Those 45 minutes for lunch were my only real freedom each day, and therefore the only real test of my resolve. We weren't allowed to take our phones into the therapy sessions, but would be given them back during breaks for practical reasons. Even then, we were encouraged to use them as little as possible. I'd nothing but my lunch money. I was also routinely tested for drink and drugs. My recovery programme wasn't just about the 8 a.m. until 5 p.m. shift in the clinic. When that was done, I would go to a Gamblers Anonymous meeting somewhere in London.

In the background, there was a lot going on. Charlotte's term was ongoing, so she had to continue going into school. The following Tuesday, after she finished work, she and Mum went back to my school to begin moving out of the flat, as it was clear that I would no longer be working there.

After my day in London, I joined them, and met the Head of HR. I informed them that I was resigning with immediate effect, which had been one of the simpler things to decide in the many hours of talking I'd done with my parents over the weekend. I told the school that I'd tried to take my own life, that I was in rehab, that it was impossible to continue in my job, and that I wanted to make things as smooth as possible. They accepted my resignation, but I had to put it in writing, which I did that night.

Before I left the premises, I collected my possessions from my locker in the staff room and from my classroom. I was accompanied – and watched closely – by HR as I did so. As I opened my locker, a heavy item came tumbling out. It was a book about the Cheltenham Festival that I'd been given by the bookmakers, Boylesports, that they had sent along with the free tickets for the festival that I'd sold a couple of weeks earlier. Perhaps they thought I had a genuine love of racing, rather than a pathological need to gamble. I'd shoved it in my locker and thought nothing of it since. And then it came thudding out. There was some gallows humour to be enjoyed on my part.

The school informed me that they had no choice but to pass the situation on to the Teaching Regulation Agency (TRA), which took the matter out of their hands and allowed them to protect the school. I was later informed that it was the first case involving gambling addiction that the TRA had ever seen. The biggest issue was my breach of data protection in contacting parents.

I could have been banned from teaching for life. While there was no doubting my wrongdoing, my addiction was taken into account. When I provided evidence of my addiction, rehabilitation, and that I was paying back all my creditors, I was cleared in the first ever case of its kind. Sadly, I fear it will not be the last.

Dad arranged a lawyer to represent me. So he spent time dealing with lawyers on my behalf while I was unable to in order to protect me, but I'd some long phone calls telling them everything, too. Letters of evidence and psychiatric assessments were required, and it was draining. It was my first experience of legal proceedings, and I was still in rehab, making it a complicated and exhausting time.

If that was arduous, it was nothing compared to contacting those I owed money to, one by one, to explain that, no, I'd not asked for money for treatment for an unwell family member or because I'd received a surprisingly hefty tax bill. Instead, I'd asked for money to fund a gambling addiction for which I was now receiving treatment.

Dealing with these responses was extremely draining. Of course, there were negative responses (mostly from the people I'd been most worried about borrowing from), but fewer than you might think. These were the conversations I'd feared so much just a few days earlier, but having them was all part of a process I was firmly committed to.

Arranging to pay back those creditors was complicated – clearly the deep shit I was in financially wasn't going to disappear overnight. In my spare time during my first week in the clinic, I contacted each person I owed money to, with a follow-up meeting in person or on the phone where necessary. In each instance I explained that I was in rehab, and that I was working out how to manage the situation.

Some of my creditors were well within their rights to sue me. For the bigger loans from savvy, high-powered businessmen, I'd been made to sign contracts (some including a witness signature, which I forged). The contracts laid out what I was borrowing, and the terms of the agreement – including what would happen if I failed to pay them back. Of course, I'd signed all these things in haste and desperation, and had not really considered the consequences, but they had every right to take me to court. Probably between £50,000 and £75,000 of my debt fell under this category, with the loans coming from around eight individuals.

Some of my other creditors explained that they needed the money back immediately, which was obviously absolutely fair enough. The same was true of Amigo Loans – I owed them around £18,000, despite keeping up with some of my repayments. For that, urgent action was clearly required, and I was fortunate that between them my parents and the Professional Cricketers' Association (PCA) – which had stepped in to help with my treatment – agreed to pay that money off immediately. I'm fully aware how lucky I was to have access to both those means.

The PCA had become involved when in a therapy session on the second day in rehab, it was suggested that we contact five people who wouldn't be aware of our new circumstances, to fill them in. It was part of the process of being honest and owning the situation we were in. With my family all in the loop, I chose five mates. I'd been dreading having to tell my friends, and I'd always thought they would ditch me if they knew what I'd become. But their reaction was so different to what I'd feared.

One of them reminded me of the PCA's help a year earlier, and suggested I get back in touch with them. I was a bit sheepish, for two reasons. First, I didn't really consider myself worthy of their help. I'd played nine first-class matches for Durham University and spent almost three years on the staff at Northamptonshire CCC, getting to the fringes of the first team before being released. I'd been a professional cricketer, but not one of note, and not for a long time. Secondly, when they helped me the year before, I had not acted in good faith.

But they were instantly keen to help more and were perhaps not totally surprised after what had happened a year earlier. While they feared gambling was prevalent among cricketers, I was the first player to get myself in this sort of mess – at least that they knew about.

They dealt sensitively with the situation, communicating a lot with my family (to make sure they were coping with the situation, too), and offered financial support for my treatment and the further counselling I received when I left the clinic after a month. These one-to-one sessions in London were important; they allowed me to talk about aspects of my recovery that I was struggling with and what I was finding hardest to adjust to and to stay on top of things. The PCA also gave me access to their Professional Development Manager for Northamptonshire as that was the county I'd played for. Each county club had one to provide support to current and former players. He gave me advice professionally, not only supporting me with building a CV and applying for jobs, but emotionally, too. They were extraordinarily generous.

I also contacted the debt management charity Step Change, who were extremely helpful. I was an unusual case because, while I had a common mix of bank and payday loan debts, I also owed significant amounts of money to many individuals. They helped set up a payment plan to all my creditors, settled monthly, based on what I could afford beyond my basic living expenses.

Paying it all off would take 14 years and three months. I then set up a separate repayment plan with my parents and the PCA, who had bailed me out with urgent payments while I was unable to earn during my rehab. As a result of setting up these payment plans, the legal cases with individual creditors were dropped. I simply can't break the agreements set now, and the threat of pressed charges and prison certainly focuses the mind when it comes to remaining on the right path.

Such a long period of repayments might sound intimidating, but it was actually a positive for me. It provided light at the end of the tunnel. When I was at my worst, I would look at the debts I'd got myself in, and see no way out apart from gambling.

Now, there was a way out. Even if the term had lasted for 40 years not 14, it will be paid off eventually. I now have to be patient and simply accept this. I view it almost like a mortgage. I don't have to commit every last penny I earn to the repayments, but for quite some time I'll have to cut my cloth and make sacrifices. Obviously at times this has an impact on Charlotte too, in the sense that we had to be very careful with our spending but were able to adapt quicker than either of us expected. In some ways, it made us appreciate what we had that bit more.

The irony is that even though I've committed myself to large monthly repayments every month for many years, I've still set myself up to have more money and income than I'd ever had because I wasn't losing money gambling.

There was an alternative path to this. I could have declared myself bankrupt and not paid any money back, but that wasn't in the spirit that I was approaching this. It would have left me with devastating consequences for much longer, and perhaps far greater legal action. I wanted to pay these people back. Not just because it made me feel better, but because I owed it to them. I wanted to show them the values that I hold when not gripped by gambling. That underneath my addiction I'm a very different person to the one who made those requests.

I handed over official management of my finances to Charlotte and my parents temporarily. I cancelled all my accounts and cut my cards up, essentially starting over to ensure total transparency with them. They were in charge for about a year as I slowly got back to my feet. For a couple of months I was totally without income and reliant on my parents and the generosity of Charlotte's family but it was not too long before I started earning again.

Amidst all this, one very good thing happened, though. On 29 March, my sister gave birth to my second niece. In a period of utter turmoil for the whole family, this was a massive positive. It did, though, make our living arrangements even more of a madhouse than they had already been. Once again, my sister had been a total hero and it was fortunate that because my parents were teachers too, we could all be together during the Easter holidays.

The birth provided particularly welcome relief for Charlotte and Mum, who threw themselves into looking after my other niece between some pretty tough conversations about my future. Charlotte and I had only been together around 18 months, and my parents had never met hers before. But the support I received from Charlotte's family was unwavering. While I was undergoing treatment, Charlotte took steps to set us up to move in with her dad and step-mother when I'd finished the first stage of my treatment, and was thinking of buying a place of her own in Oxfordshire.

Each day when I returned from the clinic I would have a queue of people wanting to discuss how the day had gone. I was drained, and some days was better at holding these conversations than others. At the weekend I would do nothing but the 'homework' we were set; and not only was I catching up on years of missed sleep, but I was going through the wringer in the week, too.

The treatment I went through was a non-residential abstinence-based programme on Harley Street in London. I appreciate how lucky I was to have access to this. The focus, in my case gambling, was to figure out what was driving it. There were about 10 of us on the programme at any one time, with a range of different addictions. I was actually the only gambling addict, which helped me hugely because it allowed me to focus on the reasons I was gambling rather than the behaviour itself. I didn't think about the act of gambling, I thought about addiction more generally.

The programme was based on Group Therapy. This approach is widely regarded as the most effective forum to treat addictive disorders. Seeing and talking to others in the same boat provides hope and confidence because however resistant and downhearted you are, you are not alone. We sat in a circle, talking and connecting our stories. This was coupled with individual therapy; two or three times each week I had a one-on-one session with a therapist. Our days were dominated by these sessions, but we also practised mindfulness, acupuncture and yoga.

There was no set time to anyone's treatment. Everyone there was at different stages of their recovery, so there was a revolving door of patients. Most people stayed for four to six weeks, and you left when you and the therapist agreed you were ready. It only worked if you wanted to be there. One bloke went for his lunch on day one and never came back.

When I went out for my lunch or headed to catch the bus home, there was temptation. I walked past betting shops and couldn't help but think about going in. I just knew I had to do the right thing, as hard as it felt. When I saw people in the shop, I didn't envy them. If anything, I worried for them.

It helped that I was broke, and excluded from any betting outlets on my phone too. It also helped that, for the first time in my life, I was disengaged from the sporting world. I had a lot going on, obviously, but I also associated sport with something I was trying to leave behind. Weekends were more of a challenge, because I particularly associated that time with sport. I sat down with Dad for a few minutes here and there to watch something but generally my mind was elsewhere and I tried to shut that world out – mainly to protect myself.

I planned my day out minutely, to leave no space for gambling. The obvious problem time was the bus home, alone. So I started writing down my thoughts for the first time ever, setting up a blog. I listened to a lot of music, which wasn't something I'd ever done much of. I also listened to podcasts that might help me understand better what I was going through. I read relentlessly about addiction. And sometimes I just slept. For the first time ever, I tried to be mindful, and looked after myself. It helped massively that I quit alcohol, too. Stopping drinking was simpler than stopping gambling. I knew it was a must in the early days of my recovery journey. After three months, I started drinking again in moderation, knowing that it was under control.

My time in rehab was excruciating. Each day was a brutal battle. At first, I was hugely cynical about what I was expected to do, and whether it could possibly work for me. But those treating me pretty quickly worked me out. They realised that, like everything in my life, I wanted a quick fix. So I was happy to talk about my thoughts, but not my feelings. I may have even thought I could be in and out in a week. But a swift resolution wasn't on the cards here. They explained that it would take much longer: there was no timeframe, and I would only be leaving when I was ready to leave. I would know when that was, they told me.

It took me at least the first week – when I was preoccupied with my thoughts about jobs, houses and money – to realise that this really would take time and to start to trust the experts. Only once I accepted that was I able to take steps forward. It had been the same for my first visit to Gamblers Anonymous (GA). I looked round a room of 25 to 30 others, from all walks of life, and thought I was nothing like those I was with. In time, I accepted that what I'd been doing was the same and, in most cases, worse. I came to understand that not every recovering problem gambler required – or was able to access – the depth of treatment I was receiving. For many, GA was the extent of their rehab.

In those first few days of treatment, I was withdrawn, crying lots and showing my anger with the world. But that was accepted – I was in an environment where showing the emotions that gambling – or lack of – made me feel was encouraged. It took a while to realise there was no judgement, and that I could embrace and express these emotions. Eventually, as I understood my addiction better, I realised opening up was therapeutic.

At the end of my third Monday in the clinic, I experienced a watershed moment. We were beginning to delve into some deep conversations, such as my relationship with my dad, and as we were about to leave, I said to Mandy, 'I'm starting to feel better.' She turned around and responded with such clarity: 'Well, we haven't even started talking about your overeating yet.' I was mortified and in complete shock that she'd said this, especially in a room full of people.

Furious, I stormed out of the clinic at the end of the day. When I got on the bus, it hit me like a wave and I burst into tears. On the way home, my mind raced through everything I'd been told over the last two weeks. Charlotte picked me up from the bus station and I was an emotional wreck, which was unusual in this situation. Normally I was drained but positive about what I was experiencing. This time, I was desperate to talk to my mum, and that evening we spoke for hours – about all sorts.

I'd always been insecure about my weight, which had ballooned. Over time I'd gone from professional athlete to a state that I was frankly embarrassed by. I knew this was a manifestation of the all-encompassing nature of my gambling addiction, and the excessive eating and drinking that went with it.

Mandy knew exactly what she was doing when she made that comment. She told me later that she'd spent a fortnight working out which buttons to push to make me crack – and it worked! It was genius. From then onwards no subject was off limits for me. They had unpicked me, and now it was time to stitch me back together.

The funny thing is, the topic of my weight never really came up again in the clinic. And I didn't suddenly stop having a complex about it. When I was finally leaving the clinic, Mandy told me that she'd previously had a patient who I was very similar to, and this technique had worked well with him. At the clinic, they spoke a lot about primary, secondary and tertiary addictions. We were trying so hard to eradicate the primary addiction – gambling, in my case – but that could result in us trying to replace it with a secondary addiction, like eating and alcohol. Mandy clearly thought I needed to be aware of that.

My development was best encapsulated by my changing attitude to *The Serenity Prayer*, which was written by the American Reinhold Niebuhr. We would say this at the beginning and end of every day and, at first, I was extremely uncomfortable holding hands with the stranger next to me and saying the simple words. It just seemed cheesy.

But as time went by, and they told us to 'trust the process' more and more, I began to understand the prayer's value, and it became important to me. It felt like the best bit of advice I'd ever been given. I had to accept that there was so much I couldn't change in my past. I had to accept the decisions *I had* made while an addict. I had to change the things that were within my power in the present and future. I could allow gambling to ruin my life forever, or I could change.

As I entered the fourth week, I realised that I was almost – not quite – enjoying myself. I felt secure, and also felt I could offer advice to people earlier in their journey. I started to feel happy, and confident that I'd done the right thing and was taking positive steps forward. I was sleeping better, which helped, but I still had low moments. The initial embarrassment wore off as I understood my illness, but shame and guilt lingered.

One of the crucial elements for me was removing the impulsive element of gambling, and I was given tools and strategies to do this. If I ever thought about gambling, or wanted to bet, rather than acting upon that impulse, I would ring or message another person in the programme to let them know. The time that took and the small act itself removed that impulse. The urges and temptations subsided just a little with each passing day, and things got easier. These were baby steps, but I could feel them beginning to work.

And they were right – I did know when I was ready to leave. Twenty-eight days is the typical rehab time and, as it happens, I was discharged at the end of my fourth week. I'm glad mine wasn't a residential clinic – it made it much easier to return to the real world. And my treatment didn't stop there. I had three more months of one-on-one counselling and aftercare sessions, and I continued going to GA sessions in Oxford at least once a week for six months. By then my life had changed considerably and I felt, for me, GA had run its course.

From the moment I came clean I never *wanted* to gamble again. But I needed to learn to deal with the *need* to gamble. That takes time, remains a work in progress and is not easy. The need would come in waves, particularly when I'd access to money, and I would have to remind myself why I was doing this and how low gambling had left me for so much of my life. The more times I batted that temptation away, the weaker it was when it next returned.

When I walked out of the clinic on 20 April, 2018, and then finished up with GA six months later, I still went to counselling, therapy and after-care sessions, which involved talking to people who'd been through the same programme, and were at different stages of their recovery. I wasn't cured. I still am not – and attend sessions whenever I feel I need to, because I'm self-aware enough to admit it. Having this outlet remains an important tool in my recovery. As a bonus, I have made lifelong friends at these sessions, who I can reach out to at any time.

By now I didn't want to gamble and was feeling much better; less fearful, and more accepting of everything I'd done. I felt like a different person and ready to get on with a new chapter in my life.

14

At the time of writing

That £100 on King Crimson in the 2.10 at Wolverhampton on Thursday 22 March, 2018, remains my last bet.

And I'm pleased and proud to say that I'm leading a very different life to the one I was when I placed it. At the time of writing, I'm well over years into a lifelong journey of recovery. It's a daily battle, but one I'm determined to win.

The first nine months of my new life were extraordinary. By Christmas 2018, having been in the depths of despair just a year earlier, I was engaged, had moved into a new house with Charlotte and stood on the threshold of a new career, which is built on preventing others making the same mistakes I did. Every really important relationship in my life had improved beyond measure.

I'd known long before things went badly wrong that I wanted to marry Charlotte but her remarkable response to my crisis only accelerated the process. She could easily have run a mile when she learnt of the situation I was in and the stream of lies I had told, but I never felt more loved and supported. She also had her world turned upside down but was a rock emotionally, and brilliantly practical too. Her family were incredible as well, offering unwavering support and no judgement. We lived with her dad and step-mother while we got back on our feet; their generosity was unforgettable.

In May 2019, we went on that trip to Amsterdam that Charlotte had given me for my birthday. It felt like a massive moment for us, a new start. I'd been out of rehab for a few weeks and I was still taking baby steps. I'd worried about how I would ever buy a ring, but my mum passed on a beautiful ring that my dad had bought to propose to her (and since replaced). On Friday 1 June, on one of Amsterdam's many bridges, I proposed. I was very relieved when she said yes!

On 18 July, 2019, we got married in front of our closest friends and family in the village Charlotte's mum lives in in Oxfordshire, before a reception in the Cotswolds. It was the perfect day, a real team effort. Charlotte worked incredibly hard preparing all sorts, while friends and family helped out with flowers, decorations and one of our great friends did an amazing job with the food. That everyone pitched in made it so much more special. It was important to us to have everyone there who had stuck by me through thick and thin over the previous 15 months. That my younger brother was my best man was extremely important to me, for obvious reasons.

My professional situation moved just as fast. The first 90 days of recovery are generally accepted to be the toughest, because of the shame and guilt, but also because you're being watched closely by all those around you. You're swimming again, but with armbands and lifeguards everywhere. I read, blogged and spoke about my addiction as I got to grips with what had happened.

From the very early days of my recovery, I was keen to share my story, not because I was proud of the turnaround I was undergoing nor because I wanted to be seen as a hero, but because I didn't want anyone else, or those around me, to go through what I did.

I wanted to shout from the rooftops about the dangers of gambling. I thought back to my own development and education. I went to elite private schools, a top university, was a professional sportsman, worked in the City and then in two schools. In the course of that journey, I was given (and gave) some vital lessons and lectures on certain issues – drinking, taking drugs and smoking. So too, eating disorders and obesity. Regrettably, it didn't stop me doing those things but I was at least aware of the dangers posed by them. But I received no education about gambling, and was totally naive to the harm it could do.

Over the course of my adult life, a sea-change was taking place. Gambling was increasingly discussed in the media, we were hearing from more problem gamblers, and the law was changing to make things safer. There was still much work to do, but people shouldn't have that gap in their education. I wanted to be part of closing it, especially for the next generation of young people.

It started with a bit of blogging and social media in the weeks leading up to me leaving the clinic in 2018. Then I needed to find work, both to keep busy and to pay the bills – and, boy, did I have some bills to pay. Initially, I managed to secure a job with a sports travel business that specialised in organising sports tours for schools. It was a good fit for me and a positive experience, starting with having to tell my story, chapter and verse, to the company's founder as part of the interview process. It was nerve-racking but cathartic. Contrary to my expectations, he didn't run for the hills. He offered me a job, which boosted my confidence no end. It made me feel accepted, wanted, and that I'd something to offer in my new self. It also reinforced my newfound belief that I should never shy away from what had gone before, or there would always be an elephant in the room.

I enjoyed the work, and was extremely grateful for it. But I also knew I wouldn't want to do it for ever. I found that, even though I was working full-time and spending so much quality time with my family and Charlotte, I now had more spare time than ever before, because I didn't have my face buried in my phone. I contacted people connected to the worlds of gambling, addiction and mental health. I thought a lot about my story and how to share it.

I soon found myself speaking at independent schools (to pupils of sixth form age) I had links to. I was beyond nervous, about how I would react emotionally to being so open so soon, about whether I could hold it together, or how I would be received. My words were raw and unpolished and I could hear a pin drop in the room as I spoke. But the reaction was warming. The talks hit home, and the feedback was positive. I got a special buzz from speaking to large audiences; it reminded me of the pressurised environment of playing cricket.

The PCA also offered me the opportunity to start telling my story in the media, and in October I was involved in the launch of the rebranded Professional Cricketers' Trust alongside Marcus Trescothick at the Oval. Marcus and I had both had our battles (his international career ended prematurely in 2006 because of depression), but he was one of England's greatest-ever batsmen, who enjoyed a 26-year professional career, whereas mine barely got off the ground. Our differences showed that the PCA would put an arm around any cricketer, no matter how illustrious their career.

I'd approached the PCA about talking to cricketers – especially those at Academy level – about my experience, and they introduced me to EPIC Risk Management, a small business they were working with on gambling education. I spoke to the founder, Paul Buck, who himself was recovering from a harrowing gambling addiction. EPIC stands for Education, Prevention, Identification, Control and its aim is to warn of the dangers of gambling.

I told him my story and said I would love to be involved. Paul was brilliant, kind and encouraging, but pointed out that I was still in the early stages of my own recovery. The basic message was that I should sort myself out before I started trying to help others sort themselves out. It was hard to argue with. Rehab had drummed into me that there could be no quick fixes here, that I was on a long journey. My instincts were for swift outcomes and resolutions and for life to be lived in a hurry, so I did need a little reining in – and it worked perfectly as a lesson in understanding the need for patience.

A few months later, as I delivered more of these talks in schools, we spoke again, and I was offered a job, initially two days a week, then full-time from the start of 2019.

There are a few strands to my job. Primarily, I deliver talks to schools. They last around an hour, with the first 25 minutes or so being a whistle-stop tour of the story that you've read in this book – how it started, the pinch points that hastened my decline, rock bottom and how I freed myself of addiction. I then highlight stats and facts about gambling, and offer some practical advice related to gambling and addiction more generally. Essentially, I try to say the words I wish I'd heard throughout my journey.

We speak at about 250 schools – both state and independent – per year, and I deliver about half of those sessions. It's vital to get into schools. There are at least 450,000 children between the ages of 11 and 16 in the UK gambling every week, 143,000 of whom suffer gambling-related harm (adverse impact from gambling on health and well-being). This has been accelerated by a convergence of video-gaming and gambling. Video games often allow users to purchase add-ons – called 'loot boxes' or 'packs' – which essentially amount to gambling, because players spend money on them without knowing what's in them. Didn't get what you wanted? Do it again. This normalises gambling behaviour for young people, and acts as a gateway drug, a sort of digital version of a scratchcard.

I also speak to professional cricketers. We work with all 18 men's first-class county clubs, both at academy and professional level, and now in women's cricket, too. I deliver these sessions with Chris Wood, a current professional cricketer who's also in recovery.

Chris has a link to another strand of my work. Fairly regularly, after one of my talks, someone will get in touch to say that they related to it, either because they're struggling with gambling, or because someone they know is. They're looking for help or advice from someone who has lived through the same thing. I'm not a counsellor and can't offer specialist treatment or support, but I can offer my own experience and guidance, gentle signposts to official help, and then an additional, anonymous support network when they do. Vitally, I can remind them that they're not alone, that there's a way out.

About six months into my job, I gave a talk at Hampshire County Cricket Club, where Chris has been an outstanding professional for more than a decade. He was actually unable to make my session because his partner was giving birth, but afterwards, he contacted me to explain that he was receiving treatment for gambling addiction, and was getting support from the PCA – as I had. We spoke lots, shared our experience and, being further along in my recovery, I was able to offer guidance. Eventually, he was ready to go public with his story, becoming the first active professional cricketer to reveal his gambling addiction. He spoke so well that soon EPIC asked if he wanted to come and work for us alongside his cricket career.

I have acted in this unofficial mentoring capacity for others, in and outside professional sport, providing gentle support and advice. There are other individuals who are getting closer to bringing their problems under control and speaking about them as the taboo around gambling addiction slowly lifts.

My work has allowed me to share my story in many different environments. We work directly with every players' association of team sports in the UK and Ireland, but also focus on other at-risk sectors such as the financial services industry, the criminal justice sector (working directly in prisons and probation teams to reduce the risk of reoffending), the armed forces and construction, among other areas.

The company has grown massively. When I started there were just half a dozen or so people involved. Now, we have almost 30 people, about half of whom have lived experience of problem gambling from all walks of life. The other half work on the coordination and management side of the business. We are working all over the UK, but increasingly in the USA and Europe, too. Our rapid growth is an indication that people are opening their eyes to the threat posed by gambling addiction.

Recovery, of course, is not a qualification to preach about gambling addiction alone, just as recovering from a broken arm doesn't make you an orthopedic surgeon. But experience is the most important tool we have, and allows us to speak with authority and empathy.

Relatability is important too, though. So I deal especially with cricket and independent schools, where I have a lot of experience, whereas my colleague Scott Davies, a former Championship footballer, deals with the football side of things. In private schools I think my background has been important; these young, privileged people who believe they're as invincible as I did and who are as naive to addiction and gambling as I was, sit up and think 'this bloke was me once'.

Generally, I think people expect us to go in and tell them not to gamble, and that they'll quickly become bored. Luckily, their expectations are usually confounded. I'm not there to tell them what to do with their lives – that would be rather rich – but to point out the dangers attached to gambling. Our method is to use our personal story, which is emotive and eye-opening. I find that people connect to my story, even when they have no relationship with gambling.

I believe that education is in my blood. I'm from a family full of teachers, grew up around schools and was drawn to the profession. I threw that career away, and very deeply regret the behaviour that led to that. So the opportunity to educate – on a subject that I never thought I would – is a real privilege. When I was gripped by addiction, I felt there was no way out, and that I was alone. Neither is true – and I want to show others that there's walking, talking evidence of that. I do have a desire to help people, I do want to be a role model, I do want to change people's perceptions of gambling, and I do feel I have societal debts to repay. But it also helps me, and makes me happy, which is a big part of why I believe it has been a success for me.

It's wonderfully rewarding work, and I enjoy mixing and talking with others who have had similar issues. I find it interesting how we all look back on our addiction slightly differently. Some feel that, for them, it could only ever have been gambling. I take a slightly more holistic view, believing that with my addictive personality I would have fallen for something, and it happened to be gambling. And just as we all have different stories of addiction, we all have different approaches to recovery. I know someone who still watches a lot of horse racing, which I just can't comprehend.

When I gambled, I was a compulsive liar, too. I learnt in rehab that recovery wasn't just about quitting gambling but all the peripheral negatives, too. Now, I'm as honest in every aspect of my life as I possibly can be. In the early days of recovery, I would still tell little lies. Charlotte would spot them immediately, and call me out on it. Slowly but surely, that need to lie has stopped.

My relationship with sport – as a viewer – has gone full circle. I now appreciate it for what it is, rather than something that I had to participate in or a means of feeding my addiction. I follow it as I did when I was a kid. I have got more into supporting the team I have supported since childhood, Liverpool, and enjoy watching all the sport I grew up watching. I appreciate the skill and tactics, rather than only caring about the outcome.

Horse racing is not on that list, though. I only got into racing – and in a pretty big way – because of my gambling. I immersed myself in it, and loved it. It's a wonderful sport, full of skill and wonderful stories. But now I don't watch or follow it, because its link to gambling is just too intrinsic and entwined. Gambling props the sport up, to the extent that many viewers forget there's anything more to it than the bets.

So I might watch the Grand National for the sporting spectacle, but nothing else. The week of the Cheltenham Festival is a painful and difficult few days each year, with the anniversary of the toughest time of my life, and all sorts of conflicting memories of the years before that. I look to counter that by renewing my push to educate people, because others will be finding that time of year tough, too.

So life is good. I'm married to a brilliant wife, have a dream job (one that I certainly never saw coming, but value dearly), and a supportive family. While I burned bridges and lost some friends with my behaviour, many more have stuck by me and I've reconnected with others through what happened, too. There are long-term financial consequences, but a very well-organised repayment plan. I have choice, motivation and am happy.

That doesn't mean it's all angels and butterflies. It's bloody tough. There's the financial element, obviously, and there are still periods of anxiety. For all the changes that have taken place, I still have the same personality – which is very susceptible to addiction.

The difference now is that I'm able to more effectively navigate the challenges I face. I found this was particularly true when issues arose for the first time after my life had changed. I can now handle bad news, whether it's receiving an email that makes my skin crawl or something more serious. Before, I always had an outlet to soften my struggles. Where once I would retreat to gambling at the first sign of adversity, I now manage and talk about my issues. I endeavour not to feel sorry for myself or curse the hand I'm dealt.

I have a self-awareness and a compassion that I didn't before. Charlotte says she saw an immediate change in how much I cared and thought about others when I came out of rehab that has grown since. She didn't know that for the first 18 months we were together, I'd so much more I could give. I'm a more helpful person who does more for those I know, because I have so much more time. The need to gamble made me selfish.

I'm aware of my shortcomings and the difficulties I face. I'd spent my whole life thrusting myself into the centre of the room because I wanted to be loved, and to be considered the best at everything – from playing sport to downing a pint in the pub. Gambling and my almost unhealthily competitive streak combined to create a wild egomaniac, built on bravado. Behind closed doors, my self-esteem was at rock bottom.

Understanding that life is not all about winning and losing has made me a kinder person. I try to extinguish, rather than spark, my ego. I can still find ways to compete – on the golf course, for instance – without causing trouble. Golf has been a great outlet, as the pace is slow and it's social. I can be competitive in a quiet and steely fashion, while also enjoying the success of the friends I play with.

I have never been good at switching off, but I'm getting better at resting my mind. As an addict, my mind moved at 100mph. I was thinking about gambling, and constantly stressed. Now everything happens more slowly. And I need to slow things down further, take my time over decisions. But I get better at it with each passing month. I'm able to relax, because I'm comfortable in my own skin.

I take my mental health seriously, and work hard on managing it, through mindfulness (using an app at the end of the day to help me switch off) and, especially, exercise. Addiction and mental health go hand in hand, because addiction so often begins as a means of coping with negative feelings or an inability to deal with issues. Certainly, that inability exacerbated my addiction and caused my mental health to deteriorate.

Back in the day, my attitude towards mental health was prehistoric. I thought silence was strength, and that talking about emotional issues was weakness. Now, I put my mental health first. If something was having a constant negative effect on my physical health, I would do something about it. If someone was making me unhappy, I would either address it with them, or see less of them. It's the same with my mental health. I know it's an issue, so I take action to address it. I'm proactive, not reactive.

My recovery has coincided with much-improved conversations in the wider world about mental health, but there's a long way to go yet. We are getting better at recognising there's an issue. The next step, I believe, is to normalise conversations about what we do to help our minds. I'm more than happy to display my vulnerability on social media and in person. Before, everything was internalised. Now, I'll share what I'm feeling or thinking.

I try to pass this message on in my role as an ambassador for a charity, the Mintridge Foundation, which aims to use sport to help young people. Their ambassadors are 'positive sporting role models' and we look to develop confidence and resilience in the kids, while teaching them the importance of their mental and physical well-being. Charity work is important to me because I spent years taking, and want to give something back.

Managing my instincts is a daily challenge. I remain obsessive and impulsive. I decided I wanted to write this book, then wrote a first draft – more than 60,000 words – in just a couple of days when the first lockdown of 2020 arrived (it's fair to say the final product that you have in your hands is rather less rushed – it took three lockdowns to write!).

I got into running – in a big way. Enjoying the mental and physical benefits, I went from struggling to run 5km (3 miles) to marathons in a matter of months. In late 2020, I ran 1,000km (620 miles) in 100 days for the Professional Cricketers' Trust, which was gruelling, but an incredible feeling. In October 2021, I ran the London Marathon, which was a very special day – and I did it quicker than I ever thought I could. I do it because it's good for my mind. That it also helps my physical health is a bonus, and I'm as fit now as I have been at any time since I was a professional cricketer.

I still drink, and often when I have two beers I want 10. I quit smoking altogether for that reason – I was never able to have just one social fag. But days of having 10 beers are few and far between where once they were habitual. I'm also constantly trying to manage my use of my phone, which became an extension of my arm when I was gambling. It's taking time to get down to a healthy screen time, but I'm making progress.

I accept this is my personality now, and work hard on it. Before it was simply a huge weakness, now it can be a strength. The challenge is to stop doing bad things and to indulge in constructive things. As I have always been, I'm a workaholic, which is a positive – in moderation. I constantly try to get things done as soon as possible and want others to operate at the same pace as me, but I'm getting better at taking a slightly more relaxed approach. The good news now is that I recognise my need for instant responses and gratification, and I have people aware of the issue to help manage it. Charlotte is very quick to spot when I need to take a step back from something.

My work presents its challenges. I spent 13 years addicted to gambling and as soon as I stopped, I kept it close at hand by surrounding myself with conversations about it. Even if I wanted to, gambling is something I can't escape because there are reminders everywhere. Every time I turn on the TV, there's an advert for some sort of gambling, from sport to bingo.

The reminders provided by advertising could – and occasionally do – make me angry, because they're so relentless, and feature deliberate hooks to draw people in – not to mention that they glamorise gambling in a way that totally distorts reality. I know they make many other people angry, including members of my family. But I have to remind myself that for every gambling addict, there are also people who have put a couple of quid on the game tonight, and will be quite happy to collect their £10 winnings without being compelled to immediately bet again. Ultimately my hope is that operators, regulators, the media and politicians do more to reduce gambling-related harm and recognise the need to work collaboratively in order to prevent people suffering in the way I did.

There's a long-term financial hangover to deal with. My repayment plan is a blessing, manageable, and I'm extremely lucky. It is, though, a shackle that prevents aspects of my life moving forward. While I earn a good living, I can't get a credit card, let alone have my name on a mortgage (Charlotte owns the house we live in). That is not to complain – as I said, I'm extremely lucky to be in this position and it keeps my recovery grounded.

I hate money and don't like talking about it. I have come full circle, from the tight teenager whose family called him a miser to the wild gambling addict who lost all sense of money's worth. I don't think I'm stingy but I don't spend money that I don't need to. It's a pleasure and privilege to be able to make a rational decision based on what I have, what I need and what I want. I monitor my spreadsheets and banking app carefully, mapping my progress in paying off each individual creditor; I have completed some, with each feeling like a wonderful achievement.

Previously I would say yes to everything, because money was irrelevant. Going on, say, a mate's stag do would have been a no-brainer. Now a big budgeting decision – and compromise – is required. But because I'm honest with people about the reasons there's no pressure. I'm not broke – I'm still able to take Charlotte out for dinner occasionally – I just use my money rather more sensibly. Rather than spending £100 on a night out in London that I was barely able to remember the following morning, I'll spend the money on something sociable and active.

I actually have an understanding of money now. I might think twice about buying a take-out espresso because I think £2.95 is a bit steep. But it's not that long since, without even thinking about it, I would have put 100 times that and more on a horse I'd never heard of called Espresso Fred in the 6.40 at Windsor on a Monday evening because my concept of money had become so warped.

One element of my recovery that I'm particularly proud of is the fact that I have not borrowed money off anyone – notably my parents – for any reason since my repayment plans were put in place. And ironically, I have more money now than I ever have, despite the depth of my debts. Charlotte jokes about how I much better I am at managing my money than she is hers, these days.

Far more difficult is managing guilt. The shame attached to my behaviour has lifted. But guilt is different, and lingers longer. I hurt and affected many people while I was gambling and feel that acutely. I have found that people have been far quicker to forgive me than I'll forgive myself. They understand that I was suffering an illness. But I still carry it with me. It's just another of the many things that keep me grounded. If I blamed anyone but myself, or there were no consequences, I honestly believe I would gamble again. But I learned the hard way that there are consequences, and they're devastating. I can't hurt those I love again.

I have been fortunate enough to be given so much in recovery by those people. My family has always been close, but now we are connected like never before. Each individual relationship has been recalibrated, and brings so much joy to my life.

I have learnt in recovery the extent of the anguish I caused my mother when I gambled. As I pushed my parents away, they knew something was up, but didn't know the extent or exactly what they were looking for. Mum and I are very similar in many ways, and she suffered physically in similar ways to me as a result of my addiction. She was so beside herself with concern that she also couldn't sleep and also suffered from a stomach ulcer. In my recovery, we speak often, and when we do it can be on a deep emotional level, and she has made a huge effort to understand my addiction and mental health. She feels like she has her son back.

With Dad, it's slightly different. It feels to us both like we are father and son again, rather than the authoritative relationship that had existed in my childhood and I forced upon him when I was older. I do not try to emulate or imitate him, I'm simply able to enjoy the things we love.

My siblings have been extraordinary, too. My sister remains a confidante, and she and Charlotte are incredibly close, too. I see her family, including their two young daughters, at every opportunity. My brother is my best mate. He had had to shoulder the shock of being on the frontline as I attempted to take my own life; he has since made a real effort to appreciate the depth and extremity of what I was going through. He has become a keen advocate of mental health awareness, too.

I mentioned earlier how wonderful Charlotte's family have been. Both sides of our families have become very close, which has been very special to watch.

All those people were rocked to the core by what they learned, and blamed themselves. The truth is that there's nothing they could have done as my condition led to self-destruction. But as I have lost my ego and edge, become more present, considerate and kind, they have learnt to trust me again.

My aim in recovery is pretty simple: to be everything that I previously wasn't, and not the lying, devious, unreliable, careless, manipulative problem that gambling addiction had made me. To have that second chance means I'm just the luckiest man alive. It is to be cherished.

15

Reflections from recovery

Recovery from addiction – an ongoing battle that never stops – is not straightforward, or without its challenges. But it is definitely possible – and it is definitely worth it. Now I have told you the story of my addiction, here are some lessons I have learnt in my recovery:

'WHAT IFS' AND 'IF ONLYS' HELP NO ONE

As comfortable as I have become recounting my life and all the mistakes I made, I don't like thinking of 'what ifs' and 'if onlys'. I don't think doing so helps me or my family. If I did, I would spend my whole life looking back, and my recovery would be impeded by questions that I'll never be able to answer.

I spent many hours in the early days of my recovery, particularly while I was having treatment, thinking about these 'what ifs'. They betray remorse and regret over the past, preventing us from living happily in the present. It can feel like an irreconcilable, futile tug of war, lamenting one minute what I should have done, then in the next minute wondering what might have been.

Of course, this doesn't mean I don't have regrets. I have thousands. And they have evolved. When I was an active addict,

I would have huge regrets about not placing a certain bet on a horse that won. Now my regret centres on the damage I caused those around me.

But all that is in my power is to repay those emotional and financial debts and come to terms with it, while rebuilding my life. It's why *The Serenity Prayer* means so much to so many of us in recovery. We can't go back and make alterations, nor can we see or control what happens beyond the moment in front of us. We can plan for the future, but we can't control it. 'If onlys' and 'what ifs' hold the power of rendering us incapable of experiencing happiness in our own reality and they rob us of being able to live the peaceful life we all crave.

If I could go back, wave a magic wand and start all over again, of course I would. But it's not an option and I can't dwell on the negatives. Wondering what we might have done differently helps no one. There are, in my opinion, much more useful questions to ask. The first is, 'Why me?' And the second is, 'What do I wish I'd known?' By exploring those questions, I feel others are less likely to follow my path.

I PUT THOSE AROUND ME IN AN IMPOSSIBLE SITUATION
My parents have struggled to come to terms with the fact that so much was going on in my life that they didn't know about, and blame themselves. They still wonder 'what if' and 'if only'.

There were red flag moments, like when I withdrew the maximum daily amount on my mum's credit card when home from uni, or required bailing out in 2016. Charlotte looks back and wonders how she didn't notice that she was living with someone placing thousands of bets every day. My siblings and friends do the same.

But the truth is that I put them in an impossible situation. I lied so much, talked my way out of things, and pushed help away. My biggest problem, in so many ways, was that I wouldn't talk honestly, and admit to needing more support.

In Mum and Dad's case, they did what any parent would have done, helping me out where possible, because their love for me was unconditional. Unfortunately, I took advantage of their kindness to the extreme, and the end result was that it enabled me to worsen my situation even further.

I can't criticise the decisions that anyone close to me took in what, for them, was an utterly unprecedented situation. They were aware something was up, but never knew the extent, because I wouldn't let them in. If they had known the true extent of my situation they wouldn't have made the same choices.

Of course, they could have taken different approaches. They could have offered me no more financial support, but I would still have found a way to secure funds. It might just have meant I reached the end of the road, and my suicide attempt, sooner.

Or they could have bundled me into the back of a van and taken me to Harley Street, demanding answers, but I wasn't ready to stop gambling until I actually stopped. Even in that scenario, I would have probably wriggled out of the straitjacket.

Perhaps most likely to work with me would have been to tell me how much anxiety and pain I was causing them, as my mum worried herself sick. All these people who cared about me, who were giving me money and signing documents on my behalf, had jobs and families that I was affecting. I only thought I was destroying myself, and insight into the collateral damage I was causing might have opened my eyes. I was so selfish, and thought I was the only one affected. But there's no guarantee this would have worked either, and it might even have pushed me to the brink through sheer guilt. It can go both ways.

The only advice I can offer is to ask, ask, and ask again. If you think something is up, be persistent but not intrusive. Attempt to comfort and coax. For some people, as I found, talking is desperately hard. For others, more direct intervention and boundary-setting might work, but there's no one-size-fits-all approach, no way of guaranteeing success.

The addict has to want to stop. Just knowing that support is available is extremely powerful. The next step is to teach everyone that recovery is possible.

I TAKE RESPONSIBILITY – BUT SO MUCH MORE COULD HAVE BEEN DONE TO PROTECT ME

I'm not proud of so much of what I did while I was an addict and carry many regrets, mainly regarding the impact of my behaviour on others. But it was all me. It was me who placed every single bet, me who told all the lies, me who caused all the trouble and me who pushed away support when it was there. I pressed the buttons, scrawled on the betting slips, typed out the emails and said the words.

But two things can be true at the same time. I take responsibility for my actions, but I also believe that there was a degree of exploitation from the gambling industry of people in my position. On a broad level, there's the relentless advertising, plastered across all sports coverage. On a personal level, think back to all those free bets, and the ease at which I was able to open all those accounts.

I used emotional blackmail to get even more out of the bookmakers, but it was only right at the very end, when I was talking about collapsed marriages, lost jobs and suicide due to my gambling, that I was shown any duty of care by the industry – and even then, not every company said anything. By then it was too little, too late. Having said that, people are often surprised to learn that I don't absolutely loathe gambling and the gambling industry. I have distanced myself from the act of gambling by remaining totally abstinent, but I have also stayed close, by working in education and around former addicts.

When delivering sessions and engaging with adult audiences, I recognise that most people can gamble without falling prey to addiction. Take my brother. We are pretty similar people – with identical upbringings and similar interests, including sport. Like me, he went to university and dabbled with gambling. But he was able to do it in a controlled fashion, in moderation, and that meant he didn't become an addict.

Most people can gamble without too much trouble, but the industry needs to protect those who are vulnerable. Much has improved since I started gambling. There's a degree of social responsibility and understanding of gambling-related harm that didn't exist then, but there's a way to go yet. While anything that is addictive is available, there will be people at risk of addiction. So society must do everything in its power to minimise that risk to as close to zero as possible. Prohibition is not the answer, because gambling is not going away.

Here are some of my own personal proposals, all of which are already in the process of being considered:

- The legal age for everything relating to gambling should rise to 18, to protect young people. This includes scratchcards and the lottery, which are legal at 16.
- Young people also need to be protected from elements of gaming (such as the lootboxes mentioned before). These allow them to engage in gambling-related behaviours, but not gamble directly. It's mixed messaging and, while it is too early to be scientifically known, many experts believe it could act as a gateway drug. There's currently no regulation at all in this area, and this must change.
- There needs to be greater focus on how much a customer can afford to gamble. More stringent affordability checks are necessary and restrictions should be automatically implemented where relevant. During my addiction I very rarely had to provide proof of funds or explain where this money was coming from (this is more common now, with gambling companies

asking for bank statements, payslips and other proof of funds). It was only when I lost astronomical amounts that anyone found out how I was funding it. This has to be done on an individual basis because what one person can afford is clearly different to another.

- We need to focus more on the time lost as well as the money. The hours spent on gambling prevent people living their lives (healthily), and time caps would be a good idea. This is especially true for online roulette or slots where the financial damage can be devastating.
- Education about the pitfalls of gambling is key to prevention, and that education needs to be funded independently of the gambling industry. As things stand, it's not. That said, it's a bonus that education is happening at all.
- Effective treatment and support needs to be accessible and readily available. Shutting accounts down or chucking people off websites is not enough of a deterrent because there's always a way round it (I should know). Proper help needs to be available – and not only for those, like me, who are privileged enough to be able to afford it. Recently the government have funded a number of NHS specialist gambling clinics, including one for young people, but not nearly enough to combat the amount that require support. While there have been improvements and additional provision in this area it is nowhere near where it needs to be and remains behind other addictions despite its alarming growth.
- VIP schemes must become a thing of the past. The gambling industry has historically rewarded people for their losses, further encouraging addicts to spend beyond their means. It takes rewarding loyal customers far too far. There's a predatory element to free bets, offers on account opening, and money-back guarantees.

It lures people in, and some are not able to step out. Many people cite introductory offers as the reason they started gambling. That wasn't the case for me, but it certainly accelerated my descent into addiction. If you need a free bet to gamble – as I did so often – you can't afford to be gambling.

- Gambling with credit of any form – I used to take out a credit card and gamble to the limit – should be impossible. We are seeing positive changes in this department, including a ban on gambling with credit cards. However, more needs to happen to stop problem gamblers accessing funds through payday lenders and other forms of credit.

I think it's fair to say that I was gambling at what I'd call the gambling industry's 'peak internet irresponsibility'. It was the advent of online gambling and betting in-play, and the regulations weren't fit for purpose in this changing world. As I write this, evidence for the first Gambling Act Review since 2005 is being reviewed, with changes hopefully afoot. It's long overdue, but hopefully some of the suggestions outlined above will be in place soon, and the vulnerable will be better protected. I'll be doing my bit to make sure they are.

THE STIGMA

I entered the world of gambling with negative preconceptions – and that stigma stuck with me. I knew nothing about it really, having not grown up around it. My family were really into sport, but two sports with a massive gambling culture, football and horse racing, weren't the hottest topics in our household. We followed and spoke about rugby union, cricket, golf and tennis much more. Obviously gambling has a big involvement in those sports, too (as I would discover), but I wasn't aware of that then.

I knew my mum thought gambling was a waste of time and money, and was against it, but beyond that I'd never had any formal education on the subject. I valued frugality, and gambling struck me as a total luxury – an activity to engage in if you didn't have to look after your money.

So from day one I felt what I was doing was naughty, dirty even. It was something I shouldn't be doing, like smoking or taking drugs. Like those things too, I was worried about what people would think of me if I was doing it too much.

Because I found gambling so enjoyable, I was doing it too much within days of placing my first bet. And so, because of my preconceptions, I told lies to protect myself and preserve the image of me as a respectable member of the stiff-lipped world I inhabited. Soon, those lies were totally out of control – along with my gambling.

That shame and stigma stuck with me throughout my time as a gambler. I came to understand that gambling was something lots of people did, but my levels were always above what would possibly be deemed 'normal'. So I kept quiet, and the taboo became around admitting I had a problem, rather than that I did it at all.

The taboo around admitting to problem gambling now reminds me of the conversation around mental health – particularly among men – a few years ago. People are struggling with it but afraid to talk, fearful about the reaction of others and how they'll be perceived. The taboo around mental health lifts that little bit more each month, which is fantastic.

I hope the same change happens with gambling, because we have a way to go. When I was going through the tough process of contacting my creditors, it was inevitable that some people would be angry, and that was fine. But a couple of reactions stuck with me. They said, 'I'm especially disappointed that it was gambling,' or words to that effect, making it sound filthy, wasteful and avoidable. I remember thinking the same of the man who I replaced in the bucket-chair at Coral in Durham all those years earlier. It's high time those attitudes changed.

THE INVISIBLE ADDICTION

After I came out of rehab I was talking to someone about my addiction and they said, 'Ah well, at least it's not drugs or alcohol,' as if it wasn't terribly serious. I found that hard to take, given what I'd experienced. It hammered home how misunderstood gambling addiction is.

It took until 1980 for problem gambling to be classed by the American Psychiatric Association as a psychiatric disorder. It was deemed an impulse control disorder, alongside the likes of kleptomania (stealing) and pyromania (setting fire to things). As recently as 2013, it was moved to the substance-related and addictive disorders category. Increasingly, neuroscience and psychology research show that gambling addiction is similar to drug addiction in the way it activates the brain's reward system, and the way in which it always demands bigger doses. We really are still getting to grips with how serious and nasty this is for the human brain.

I wouldn't wish to rank and rate addictions from least to most unpleasant. And I wouldn't want to compare or contrast addictions with other mental health struggles. It's futile. They're all awful. They all do things to you that others don't. Gambling addiction's super-strength – the thing that makes it quite so corrosive – is that it can be so easily masked. Unlike nicotine, alcohol or drug addiction, there is no obvious physical change for those around the addict to pick up on, as my case illustrates. I put on lots of weight, but could easily blame that on all sorts (particularly my secondary addiction to alcohol). There's no physical limit to the amount you can gamble, unlike addiction to alcohol or drugs – you can just keep feeding your addiction until the money runs out. As I proved, a desperate mind can be extremely resourceful – and devious – when it needs money to feed an addiction.

THERE'S NO TYPE... BUT SOME OF US ARE MORE VULNERABLE THAN OTHERS

Having believed that I was totally alone while in the eye of the storm, I have since met hundreds of gambling addicts. And the main thing that has struck me is that there's no type. When I walked into my first GA meeting – when I met other gambling addicts for the first time in my life – I was taken aback. All these people have a problem with gambling? No way.

Whatever your preconceived ideas are about what a gambling addict looks like, it's so much broader than that. We come from a wide range of backgrounds, do it for a range of different reasons, and gamble on all sorts of things. There are those who gamble because they have too much money, and those who gamble because they have too little. There are those who do it for a dose of escapism, and those who need that rush. There are those who love sport, and those who have never placed a sports bet in their life.

You just need to look around the recovering addicts I work with. Three of us have a background in professional sport – a cricketer, a footballer and a rugby player. Others have worked in HR, manufacturing and the gambling industry. Another was into gaming, and slot machines, and never touched a sports bet. We are all very different, but bound by our addiction to gambling.

However, there are certain people who are more at risk than others. At EPIC, my past career makes me quite useful. Our research shows that the six highest risk sectors for gambling addicts are: professional sport, education (students, at school or university), the gambling industry, criminal justice (those in prison), financial services and the armed forces. It's extraordinary, really, that I was ensconced in three of those industries by the age of 25 as a student, cricketer, insurance broker and teacher. And for much of that time, I was indeed an addict.

The risks in the education sector (particularly to those at university), and the financial services industries, speak for themselves, I think. We need to make young people aware of the dangers gambling poses, not least because their departure from the education system broadly coincides with the moment it becomes legal for them to gamble. It's almost a rite of passage to try a beer, a smoke, a punt, even drugs, before you leave school. There's no mistaking the dangers of the others, but gambling is underestimated. For so many, like me, addiction begins at university, when we are impressionable, time-rich, free from parental supervision and have access to funds through a student loan.

Those who work in finance are vulnerable for a few reasons. They're normally paid well, and have plenty of disposable income. This means they can have significant gambling issues that remain invisible, because of the resources available to them. Risk-taking and gambling can be wrapped up in the very nature of their job, and are often embedded in the social scene.

Sportspeople are also particularly vulnerable:

- **The buzz**. Sportspeople are always looking for ways to replicate the buzz their chosen sport gives them. That dopamine hit, that euphoric feeling that comes with scoring a goal or, in my case, taking a wicket.
- **Competitive nature**. Often the sheer will to win is a major driver of their success. Those who simply love to win are more likely to bet again after a loss.
- **Time**. Sportspeople work on different schedules to most people, and it normally involves a lot of downtime. They train, but not all day, every day. They have an off-season, which often lasts weeks. They spend time on coaches and in hotels, away from home. And injuries are an inevitable part of the job, which means more time with little to do. Boredom is a major catalyst for gambling addiction, and top-level sportspeople can often find themselves bored.
- **Knowledge**. Working in sport can lead to a belief that you know more than the average punter and are more likely to win.

- **Escapism**. A high-profile day job in a brutal results business – with media scrutiny, contract pressures and injury woes – can require an outlet and escape. Gambling can appear a 'healthy' form of escapism – you don't fail a substance test when you do it, and it doesn't directly impact on your physical health like drink, drugs or smoking might. As I demonstrated, there can be no visible signs for years.
- **Money**. Sportspeople tend to have access to disposable income, and can be financially driven. Young players see older players on bigger contracts and want to make it there – fast.
- **Young and impressionable**. A desire to be accepted and be part of the changing room. The feeling of getting a new contract or big new deal is also not dissimilar to having a big win while gambling. This also adds to the financial side because they then have even more money to gamble with, which in turn fuels a desire to do it again.
- **Normalisation**. Their work uniform has a gambling logo on it, the league they play in is sponsored by gambling, their employer is sponsored by gambling and, in some individual sports, the players themselves are sponsored by gambling. It's totally normalised.

Almost every single one of those points applied to me, and that's before all the changes we've seen since my time as a professional. You only have to look on Instagram to see the amount of time our sportsmen spend online gaming (which has only increased during the pandemic lockdown and the bubbles in which they played during that time), and what I previously mentioned about the way the two are linked.

GAMBLING IS DEFINITELY NOT JUST A MALE PROBLEM
I, like many people, believed that gambling was a problem only really affecting men. My experience was synonymous with

so many male traits – particularly a powerful ego. In my early gambling days I spent hours in betting shops and casinos almost exclusively populated by men. I very rarely came across women.

I know now that there are thousands of female problem gamblers – and the numbers are increasing at an alarming rate, in fact, quicker than those of men. It would be easy to assume that their experiences are different to men's, but there are similarities. The advent of online gambling has meant that it's now acceptable in so many guises. An example of this is the way a game like Bingo has been redefined, with its advertising clearly targeting the female population.

I can't speak directly for other addicts, but to illuminate this issue, a fellow recovering addict was brave enough to share her experiences with me. Knowing her story as I do, there were numerous similarities in that it began at university, included an early big win, and resulted in huge amounts of unsustainable debt that led to actions she would regret forever. But there were also some differences, both in how she gambled and its mental toll. She says:

> *In my opinion, gambling addiction is very different for women but the repercussions of gambling addiction and the outcome or lasting effects at the end of an addiction are exactly the same. I think that with men there's a toxic culture, that gambling is normalised in college/university, workplaces and sports events. For instance, if a man tells their friend that they've just spent £200 betting on a horse that they couldn't afford to lose it'll be joked about and not seriously discussed. Whereas with women there's no discussion, whether that be a 'good' or 'bad' discussion about gambling.*
>
> *I gambled mostly on online slots (which I knew having worked in the gambling industry). At first, I'd stake around £1 or £2 per spin but sometimes this would escalate to £50 or £100 per spin. At times I had gone into bookies, but I think*

because it's a very male-orientated environment it pushes a lot of women (including myself) to gamble online instead.

I have had conversations with women about gambling. While I was working in the industry it tended to be that a lot of the customers' husbands, partners and children were unaware of their gambling. There were times they would purposely stay in the shop and 'hide' because family members had walked past and they didn't want to be seen. It also tended to be that shop gambling was a way for most women to socialise.

Since coming clean about my gambling I have had conversations about female help and support, mainly due to the idea that GA meetings tend to be all-male. Perhaps there should be women's-only GA groups, to help women feel more comfortable opening up.

More women (and men) are coming forward and telling their story. The more people who do that makes it easier for those struggling with addiction to realise it can and does get better. It's never too late to get help! Whether your problem gambling has just begun or you've been dealing with your addiction for 10 or more years, change is always for the better. The key to my recovery was being honest and open with everyone.

IF IT CAN HAPPEN TO ME, IT CAN HAPPEN TO ANYONE – GUARD AGAINST COMPLACENCY

I grew up thinking issues like addiction couldn't affect me, because I was privileged and untouchable. I had had no education about gambling, but when I heard talks about addiction to alcohol or drugs, I always thought this was something that didn't happen to people like me. The people telling the stories – however compelling the story, and however well they were telling it – tended to have come from a more challenging background, or suffered shocking trauma in their lives that set them off on a path to using addictive substances. Neither of these applied to me and, in my mind (and I believe the minds of many others in similar situations), I was therefore the least likely person to become an addict, and to end up doing the shameful things I did.

That complacency to the dangers of addiction and that ignorance of gambling addiction were among my biggest failings. When I became an addict, I refused to accept that it was happening, or that it would get that bad – until it had, and by then I believed there was no way out. I want to break down barriers and show that addiction doesn't discriminate.

I grew up with every advantage in life. There was never any shortage of love and support in my happy, close family. During my time at boarding schools and a top university, I was popular, successful and happy. I was always sociable and made friends easily, and that stretched into adulthood.

Growing up, while cash wasn't unlimited, I never went without. During my education, I mixed almost exclusively with people from similar privileged backgrounds – and some who were extremely wealthy. From the moment I left school, I had access to more cash than I needed, because I was paid to be a sportsman. After that, my jobs in the City and two schools saw me surrounded by people with plenty of money. I had always been around wealth.

I took advantage of the privilege brought by my family, friends and financial situation. I exploited individuals' means and generosity to keep my addiction alive. Had I not been in such a fortunate position, I believe my gambling addiction would have been revealed much sooner, either because I would have been caught breaking the law, or because I would have attempted to take my own life more quickly.

My background and the success I experienced as a youngster perhaps led me to believe I was bulletproof and others to consider me strong, and not vulnerable. From the outside, I looked like I had everything I could have wanted. I compounded that by putting on a facade as a confident character who was indestructible.

I also piled pressure on myself to uphold the standards I believed were expected of me in every aspect of my life. It was obviously unsustainable, and the second things went wrong, I desperately needed an outlet. That pressure also led to sneaky behaviour becoming habitual as I put on a front to maintain my image.

My privilege also played a big part in my recovery. That loving family have stood by me through everything and, with the help of the PCA, we were able to afford private rehabilitation that set me on the path that I remain on today. I'm well aware of how fortunate that makes me.

THE PANDEMIC? WHO KNOWS

The expansion of the company I work for is an indication that gambling is a growing problem. We might all be ever more aware of the issues, and things might be improving in some ways, but I also believe we've never needed to be more on our guard.

As with so many areas of our lives, the impact of the Covid-19 pandemic and its punishing lockdowns on incidences of gambling addiction is not yet clear. But what we can be sure of is that the risk factor has risen. People have faced an extended period of isolation, boredom and, in many cases, financial pressure. They have seen their families less. Their regular leisure and entertainment activities – whether that is socialising in a pub or playing sport – have not been available.

One thing that has remained available is gambling – even when there was no sport on. Online slots, casino and bingo (which is contributing heavily to rising rates of gambling addiction among women) were still there (and advertised heavily on the screens we spend all day staring at), and their high-frequency nature and accessibility make them extremely addictive and potentially destructive.

If I was to look at my crystal ball, I suspect that addictions to gaming and social media will join gambling in becoming a hot topic over the next few years. They provide the same instant response and gratification (in social media's case, through 'likes' and interaction). The younger generation has grown up hooked, and nothing is being done about it.

WE ARE AT OUR MOST VULNERABLE AFTER A BIG WIN

One common connecting thread among the compulsive gamblers I have met is the big early win. Winning almost £35,000 on that innocuous December evening in London was my point of no return. I'd been gambling for four years and with increasing aggression, but this took me to a whole new level, and it made me believe that a big win like that would happen again at any time.

When I look at the 'what ifs' – there's one. With that amount of money, and on my City salary, I could have bought myself a tidy house in my mid-20s. Now I'm in my mid-30s and unable to get a mortgage because of the damage caused by my gambling.

People usually react in two ways after a big win. Some people are able to withdraw the money, keep it in the bank or use it to improve their life. The next time they place a bet, it's with their usual little stake. The big win doesn't change their behaviour, just their bank balance. They appear to be the minority and if you're one of those lucky few – good luck to you.

Far more common is the situation like mine, where there's a constant attempt to replicate the big haul. The result is a loss of all the winnings – and then some. Some people do fall between those extremes, keeping some money, but upping their stakes a little. But that is still dangerous – the winnings are soon likely to be at risk.

Big wins come in different shapes and sizes. By the time mine arrived, I was already a habitual gambler used to winning hundreds. The step to winning tens of thousands was always likely to be disastrous. For others, winning a couple of hundred quid might seem stratospheric, and enough to completely change habits.

The big win sustains you. It provides a new benchmark and creates a belief that this is normal, and is bound to happen again. When you're in financial trouble, you look back to that moment when you won big and see replicating that as a route to salvation. I *expected* to win big again.

I try to educate people on this in any way possible. It's commonplace on social media for gambling accounts with hundreds of thousands of followers to share an image of Joe Bloggs' extraordinary accumulator, from which he has taken home thousands from a £2 stake, or similar. If I see this, I'll often reply to the person who has won, congratulating them and reminding them to raise a glass – but also warning them to take care, and withdraw the money from their online account (as I should have done).

Normally, I get a load of replies from others calling me a 'melt' and a 'killjoy', and telling me that I must be fun at parties. But I really believe in this, and will keep doing it in the hope that the message gets through, to even one person.

The biggest win available? Walking away.

LOSING CAN BE ADDICTIVE TOO

I can't easily put into words the feeling that gambling gave me. What I can explain, though, is the fact that, for me, the anticipation became more important than the outcome. Long before I placed my first bet, I'd always loved winning at whatever I was doing. I considered winning to be almost tantamount to a character trait – I was a winner. I was addicted to it. Hand in hand with that comes the fact that I was a poor loser, especially as a child. I hated losing, and feared failure. The standards I set myself in competitive educational environments meant that failure and losing were horrible thoughts.

When I discovered gambling, the rush of winning provided me with a state of total euphoria that I wanted all the time. I kept chasing that.

But that feeling was so special in part because it was preceded by another even more intoxicating sensation: the adrenalin rush I would get from waiting to find out if I'd won or lost. The suspense of the ball-bearing circling the roulette wheel, the minutes waiting to see who would score first, or the sparring as the horses ran sent my heart and mind racing.

Other gambling addicts are different, and for some of them it's all about the result – the winning and the losing. But for me, it was about the wait for the unknown outcome. Perhaps that made me even more susceptible to addiction, because losing was moreish too. I also found that losing wasn't the disaster it might seem, because it made the feeling of winning that much sweeter. My response to losing, which I considered a failure, was to try to put it right as soon as possible.

Loving the process more than the outcome was certainly a recipe for an expensive addiction, because only a complete lack of funds could actually stop me going back for more. And as I've showed, I would go to extreme lengths to ensure that I didn't go bankrupt.

The more I gambled, the more I thought this way, and the more my desire to actually win dulled. That might explain why, when I was unable to watch a race live, I wouldn't just check the result, but scour through liveblogs, following the action as it had happened, keeping that suspense alive. It was all about having a dog in the fight. And gambling gave me that on tap.

ALWAYS CHASING THE FEELING PROVIDED BY THE VERY FIRST WIN

I spent 13 years trying to top the feeling of the first bet I ever placed when, with such low expectations and a hangover at Coral in Durham, the green zero came good for me on the roulette wheel. Try as I might, I never could replicate that sense of euphoria, that instant gratification. Had I gambled for another 100 years, I never could have.

Perhaps the buzz I got from the wait for the outcome was so pure because I believed that each bet would be the one that bettered the first one I ever placed. It never was – even the big win that changed my life.

YOU ONLY EVER HEAR ABOUT THE WINS

When you hear about gambling in the media it strikes me that you only ever hear about the wins. You'll see those posts on Twitter or articles in the papers or websites about a certain remarkable win. Occasionally you'll see one where the bet has not come through, but that is only ever when the stakes have been low and the odds outrageous. A small loss on an outrageous shot.

That's because people never talk publicly about their losses. Why would we? We don't tend to boast about our disappointments. But the reality is that there's far more losing going on in gambling than winning; the cliché is that the bookmaker always wins, and there's a reason the gambling industry is in such rude health (Bet365's Chief Executive took home Britain's biggest ever salary, of £421m, in 2020).

The upshot of people only sharing their wins is that those who do not gamble – say you're an impressionable 17-year-old on Twitter – see these outrageous wins as commonplace and attainable, because they're not seeing both sides of the coin. There's now a strong community in recovery trying to work against this culture by telling the other side of the story. But we remain a very small minority.

It's the same in real life. When I gambled, there were mates I talked gambling with. But they thought I gambled at similar levels to them. At first that's because I would only ever mention the wins. Later, when my stakes were out of control, I would hide from them how much I was gambling.

The internet was a minefield, too. I was so desperate to gamble that I followed every tipster I could find, poring through articles for information on the subject of my bets. I would see one tipster had said one thing, and another a completely opposing view on the same race or game. I would end up putting bets on both and neither would win. And guess what? I would never tell anyone about that loss.

One of the reasons I felt so alone while gambling was because everything else I saw online about gambling suggested that everyone else was winning, while I was losing. Of course, this wasn't true, but it was the warped view I felt. It made me feel even lower about my fortunes.

Gambling should never be viewed as a means of making money (although clearly some people always will, including professionals), but a mere form of entertainment.

IT'S IRREPLACEABLE – BUT THAT'S OK
The plain truth is that, in recovery, I can't replace the dopamine hit that gambling gave my brain. Nothing can fill that void, because it was so pure, so instant, and so readily available to me. There are things that come close, but nothing can replace gambling.

I have, though, found ways to make up the shortfall and get that buzz in healthier quantities. As my ego has reduced, so has my demand for those thrills that I used to crave. My reconnection with the innocent joy of sport has helped, both watching and playing. The feeling of finishing a run comes close, so does taking a wicket when I play cricket. And my job is crucial to this, too. It's a real thrill finishing a talk, hearing people react to my story and, hopefully, helping others.

In recovery, I get my buzz in a very different way. I get it from things that cause me to stop and consider, rather than wait in anticipation. I get it from things that remind me how I'm rebuilding my life. That might be the feeling at the end of a run, or another sporting pursuit.

There's a temptation to gamble again, because the feeling that it gave me was so special and it was such a big part of my life. Initially, I felt a tinge of jealousy when I was reminded of others – the majority – who were able to gamble in moderation. Part of me wished it was me.

But that temptation and jealousy dies inside me a little more each day. What keeps me on the straight and narrow is the knowledge that if I relapse, I'll lose so much. Ultimately, I would likely end up in prison or dead. I have proved that once already – I do not need to again. The lows so emphatically outweigh the highs that I know it's not worth even a moment's thought.

REDEMPTION

When I do my talks, I have a number on the opening slide. It's the number of days since I last placed a bet, and my life changed. It's well into four figures now, and updating it is a daily reminder of the progress I'm making, one small step at a time.

In the community of recovering addicts, anniversaries and milestones are celebrated heartily. I make a big deal out of my friends' and colleagues' big days, and they do the same for me. The tendency is to celebrate the earliest ones hard because it does get easier and the years do seem shorter, the deeper you get into your second life.

It's a moment to thank all those who have helped you. It's a reminder of all the hard graft that has gone into getting as far as you have, and of everything that is so much better now than it was before. For me, that means literally every aspect of my life. There's nothing I would trade for one more bet.

As you'll know from this book, my date falls in March. It's close to my birthday, close to my niece's birthday, and close to the Cheltenham Festival. I can't deny that it's a tough month full of awkward memories and complex emotions, especially as the Festival is such a popular and high-profile event.

One year felt an incredible achievement. The first reminder of anything important does. I couldn't believe it was a whole year, and my life had changed beyond recognition. If I was to pick one out, though, it would be my third anniversary. That felt significant because on my second, the UK was placed into lockdown. After a torrid year and the longest winter, we were only just emerging from the latest stint in lockdown when my third anniversary rolled around.

The pandemic presented a mortal threat to my recovery. As it was for so many people, it posed an intimidating challenge. Many of the building blocks my recovery relied on, such as seeing family, were taken away for much of the year, and I had to adapt to a new way of living and working. In the past, that would have derailed me, and I would have thrown myself headlong into gambling. Had this happened in my first year of recovery even, I dread to think what would have happened.

But I coped, and made it to that third anniversary without cause for alarm, feeling proud as punch and stronger than ever. It had been a reminder to take each day at a time, and not become too consumed with the future. If I keep doing that, the next anniversary will arrive in no time.

I have a memento that I keep on my bedside table, given to me by the clinic when I was discharged. It's a heart-shaped stone with the words 'Be Kind' carved into it. Everyone gets one with a different message when they leave and, although it's a bit cheesy, it really struck a chord with me. That phrase is bandied around on the internet these days and has perhaps lost a bit of its value, but it's advice to live by. I have been so much kinder to myself and to others than I ever was before.

The tokens, anniversaries and numbers are great, but it's the little unexpected things that really hammer home how far I have come. Each bit of progress at work. Each bit of adversity handled better. Each unexpected curveball negotiated. Each old friend who gets in touch to rekindle our relationship after time apart.

Perhaps most magical of all has been each bit of support offered to someone struggling, and each creditor paid off in full.

That has happened a few times now, and is a special feeling. I love checking my financial spreadsheet to monitor my progress, even if I'm still only in the foothills of that particular mountain.

In spring 2021, one of the people I'm slowly but surely paying off got in touch with a question that took me by surprise. He asked if I would be interested in a gig coaching his kids cricket over the summer. Even though so many of them have been wonderfully understanding, my default position is to assume that all my creditors loathe me. They have good reason to. Not only did I dupe them into giving me money, but I became a pretty shoddy teacher of their kids, too.

So I couldn't quite believe what I was reading. I said to Charlotte, 'Surely he can't stand the thought, let alone the sight, of me?' 'Clearly not,' she replied. It was a reminder that people do forgive and understand. It was an honour to be asked, and I was delighted to accept the offer.

At around the same time, another nice cricket-related thing happened. I'd stayed in touch with a couple of the lads at Horspath, the club I'd represented for years but badly let down at the peak of my addiction. One of them said that if I wanted to, I'd be more than welcome to return to the club as a player or a coach. I mulled the decision over and got in touch with a lot of people at the club to make sure I wouldn't be putting noses out of joint if I did come back. But all of them were so welcoming, and soon there was a lovely article about me on the club's website as they announced the news. It was very special, and I feel quite emotional about the whole episode. It's so good to be back.

My talks provide me with a daily reminder of how far I have come. Shortly before my dad retired, I gave one at a conference of almost 200 headteachers, where he was in the room. It was brutal for him, and tough for me, but he listened throughout. His reaction and the pride I saw meant so much.

At the other end of the spectrum, I have spoken at schools that kids I once taught have moved on to. Many of them are aware of my situation, but their reaction – the sheer disbelief etched on their face – when they hear my story is very powerful. In a couple of cases they have gone back to tell their parents, who I owed money to, and they have got in touch to say well done. It will not repair the damage caused, but the pieces are being picked up.

Each little second chance like this makes me so happy that I have been given the big second chance that I'm now living. Another brick laid in my rebuilt life. Addiction left me feeling totally disheartened and bereft, behaving like a madman, and letting everyone I knew down. I thought there was no way out. Even in the early days of recovery, the shame was so deep that I didn't believe I would ever feel confidence and self-worth again.

That fog is lifting and, while I know that there's still pain as well as joy to come, with the support of Charlotte and my family, I'm ready to take it on. Already, I have achieved so much that I thought was impossible, and if even one person is helped by me, or understands addiction better as a result of the message I share, then I'm happy.

It has been a horrible road to get here, one I wouldn't wish on my worst enemy. There were so many negatives along the way, but positives have emerged. I do not believe I was ever a bad person, but addiction made me do awful things and behave in an awful way. It doesn't excuse me, but might provide context. Regardless, recovery has made me a much better person than the one who became an addict. I value what matters now.

I know that so much of what I did as a gambler can't be fixed, and that I'll carry some of the consequences with me forever. It devastates me and I wish none of it had happened. But I'm at peace with that, because I also know that there's so much living left to do, so much I can put right. And, having started at rock bottom, that is plenty good enough for me.

REFERENCES

Chapter 1

UK and international research has found that 4–11 per cent of
suicides are related to gambling, equivalent to 250–650 deaths per
year in the UK.

*Gambling with Lives – Supplementary written evidence (GAM0131),
7 April 2020.* https://committees.parliament.uk/writtenevidence
/2093/pdf/

Chapter 2

In a study regarding university students' gambling, it was found that
47 per cent of students have gambled in the past 12 months, of
which 16 per cent are moderate risk or problem gamblers.

Hodge, S. (2019). How gaming & gambling affect student life. YGAM.
https://www.ygam.org/wp-content/uploads/2020/07/FINAL
-research_full_report-PRINT-READY-5.pdf

Chapter 3

Professional sportsmen and women are three times more likely to
develop a gambling addiction. https://www.thepca.co.uk/press-
release/new-research-shows-sports-gambling-problem/

Chapter 4

A large contemporary UK study found participation in gambling in
the last year was reported by 54 per cent of 17-year-olds, rising
to 68 per cent at 20 years, and 66 per cent at 24 years, with little
overall variance. Six to 8 per cent of females and 13–18 per cent
of males were regular weekly gamblers, and patterns of regular
gambling appeared to be set by the age of 20 years.

Hollén, L., Dörner, R., Griffiths, M.D. et al. *Gambling in Young Adults Aged 17–24 Years: A Population-Based Study. J Gambl Stud 36, 747–766 (2020).* https://doi.org/10.1007/s10899-020-09948-z

Chapter 5

There are associations between problem gambling and mental health (anxiety, neurotic symptoms and substance use problems) and psychosocial maladjustment (suicidality, financial difficulties and social support).

Cowlishaw S and Kessler D. (2016) Problem Gambling in the UK: Implications for Health, Psychosocial Adjustment and Health Care Utilization. Eur Addict Res. 22(2):90-8. doi: 10.1159/000437260. Epub 2015 Sep 8. PMID: 26343859.

Chapter 6

Thirty-four per cent of gamblers say that adverts prompted them to gamble. Free bets or money to spend with a gambling company were the most likely to prompt a customer to engage with gambling. https://igamingbusiness.com/gambling-commission -customers-say-ads-prompted-gamble/

Chapter 7

Every problem gambler directly affects at least 10 other people. With 450,000 problem gamblers in the UK, there are 4.5 million people negatively affected by gambling addiction.

Productivity Commission 2010, Gambling, Report no. 50, Canberra https://www.pc.gov.au/inquiries/completed/gambling-2010/report

Chapter 8

'Higher gambling is associated with a higher rate of using an unplanned bank overdraft, missing a credit card, loan or mortgage payment, and taking a payday loan. A 10 per cent increase in absolute gambling spend is associated with an increase in payday loan uptake by 51.5 per cent. And the likelihood of missing a mortgage payment [increases] by 97.5 per cent.'

Muggleton, N. et al. (2021). *The association between gambling and financial, social and health outcomes in big financial data. Nat Hum Behav 5, 319–326* https://doi.org/10.1038/s41562-020-01045-w; https://www.ox.ac.uk/news/2021-02-04-oxford-gambling-study-fun-can-stop-financial-problems-addiction-unemployment-ill

Chapter 9
Gambling addiction is estimated to cost the UK up to £1.2 billion per year.
Finder (2020) *Gambling statistics 2020: Learn more about how Brits gamble.* https://www.finder.com/uk/gambling-statistics

Chapter 10
Numerous studies have found a relationship between problem gambling and crime, including fraud and forgery.
Lind, K. et al. (2015). *From problem gambling to crime? Findings from the finnish national police information system. Journal of Gambling Issues, 30, 98–123.* doi:10.4309/jgi.2015.30.10

Chapter 11
The average age of someone who dies from suicide due to gambling harm is 47. People with gambling problems are twice as likely to die from suicide compared to the general population.
Public Health England (2021). *Gambling-related harms evidence review: the economic and social cost of harms*

Chapter 12
In 2020, 58 per cent of 11–16-year-olds saw or heard gambling adverts or sponsorship, of which 7 per cent said this had prompted them to gamble when they weren't already planning to.
Gambling Commission (2020). *Young People and Gambling.* https://www.gamblingcommission.gov.uk/news-action-and-statistics/Statistics-and-research/Levels-of-participation-and-problem-gambling/Young-persons-survey.aspx

Chapter 13

Over £600 million is spent on betting at the four-day 2020 Cheltenham Festival.

Freebets (2020) Cheltenham Festival 2020 – Interesting Fun Facts & Figures. https://www.freebets.com/horse-racing/cheltenham-festival-betting/cheltenham-festival-2019-interesting-fun-facts/

Chapter 14

Despite the severe consequences, many individuals suffering from a gambling disorder have been reported to abstain from seeking treatment.

Håkansson, A., & Ford, M. (2019). The General Population's View on Where to Seek Treatment for Gambling Disorder – a General Population Survey. Psychology research and behavior management, 12, 1137–1146. https://doi.org/10.2147/PRBM.S226982

Chapter 15

Around 14 per cent of gambling addicts experienced at least one relapse during therapy and the subsequent follow-up.

May-Chahal, C. et al. (2017) Gambling Harm and Crime Careers', Journal of Gambling Studies, 33(1), pp. 65–84. doi: 10.1007/s10899-016-9612-z.

Echeburua, E. et al. (2001). Predictors of therapeutic failure in slot-machine pathological gamblers following behavioural treatment. Behav Cogn Psychother, 29:379-83.

Gomez-Pena, M. et al. (2012). Correlates of motivation to change in pathological gamblers completing cognitive–behavioral group therapy. J Clin Psychol, 1–13 https://www.greo.ca/Modules/EvidenceCentre/Details/what-do-we-know-about-relapse-pathological-gambling

ACKNOWLEDGEMENTS

Neither this book nor my ongoing recovery from crippling gambling addiction would have been possible without the support I have received. There are so many people and organisations I would like to thank, and it is important that I do. I will inevitably forget someone – and my genuine apologies if that is you – but the list is endless.

First and foremost, I would like not only to thank but to dedicate this book to my amazing wife Charlotte, my mum, my dad, and my brother and sister. Charlotte has been nothing short of incredible. She is a truly amazing person. It would have been so easy for her to walk away, but she didn't. For that I owe her everything. My family's unwavering support and unconditional love has been nothing short of extraordinary. I cannot express how much I love you all.

My wider family members and my long-suffering in-laws have also been with me every step of the way. Thank you.

Going through challenges like mine reveals who your true friends are. To all of you, I am so thankful to you for sticking by me and being there for me through thick and thin.

To Mandy Saligari and the incredible team at Charter Harley Street: thank you. I have said it before, and I will say it again: those four weeks transformed and saved my life.

The support of the Professional Cricketers' Association (PCA) and Professional Cricketers' Trust (PCT) were instrumental in my early recovery, allowing me to get my own two feet back on the ground and kick-start my life again. Both organisations make a life-changing difference to professional cricketers, both past and present.

It would be remiss of me not to mention all those people I let down through my addiction. To those creditors who have afforded me their forgiveness and in so many cases provided me with support: I will never forgive myself for what I did, but your response and understanding said a lot about the people that you are.

My sincerest gratitude to Paul Buck (CEO and Founder at EPIC Risk Management) for believing in me and giving me the opportunity and platform to use my experiences and do what I do now. Thank you to all the team at EPIC for their ongoing support and friendship and to my biggest ally in recovery, Scott Davies, for keeping me grounded and being there for me 24/7.

I am very proud to be an ambassador at The Mintridge Foundation. It is humbling that I now use my experiences to inspire and educate young people. To Alex and the all the ambassadors, you are a very special group of people, who inspire not only me but everyone you come across.

There are a number of people who made special contributions to this book who are much more high profile than me – your support means everything. Special thanks to Marcus Trescothick for his foreword. Thanks to all who have endorsed the book or supported it in any way.

It has been an enormous pleasure to work with Charlotte, Zoë and all the team at Bloomsbury, including Will's sister Katherine. Their enthusiasm for my story, professionalism and judgement have made this book possible. Thank you also to David Luxton for his work in getting the project off the ground and giving us a shot.

Finally, to Will Macpherson, who made this dream a reality. Not only is Will a great friend, but also a very talented journalist and writer. He has managed to articulate my story and has enabled me to put everything I wanted to down on paper in a compelling and powerful way. Thanks for putting up with me through all those Zoom calls during lockdown and my barrage of WhatsApp messages and voice notes.

My warmest and most heartful thanks to each and every one of you. As much as I would love to go back and change the past, I can't. But what I am determined to do is to start where I am and change the future and the ending. I owe that to you all.